"*Unfailing Love* offers a rich, e[...] care rooted in the unwavering [...] of devotions doesn't shy aw[...] dementia; instead, it meets the[...] [...], interweaving honest expressions of lament with unshakeable hope. Each reflection creates a sacred space where caregivers are invited to find themselves held within God's steadfast love. This is more than a devotional—it's a compassionate companion, embracing the complexity of dementia with theological depth and pastoral gentleness. *Unfailing Love* honours the dignity of all involved, reaffirming that even amid dementia's fragmentation, the God who knows us fully remains present, steadfast and loving."

> **Rev. Professor John Swinton,** Professor in Practical Theology and Pastoral Care, University of Aberdeen; Author, *Dementia: Living in the Memories of God*

"I'm delighted to commend these Bible meditations and, at times, heart-rending personal testimonies, not least because my dear father suffered an accident which vastly accelerated the decline of his mind. I watched first-hand as my family and a number of other carers sought to look after him in the midst of dementia. Strikingly, the two best carers he had were sustained by a radiant Christian faith, and it really did make a huge difference in the long hours of caring for my father. So it's a privilege to recommend this book, which helps to sustain those who are undertaking this incredibly challenging calling."

> **Rico Tice,** Founder, Christianity Explored Ministries

"This poignant book offers a lifeline of hope and comfort to dementia caregivers. Through its tapestry of bite-sized biblical reflections interwoven with real-life stories, it provides much-needed solace and reminds caregivers that they are not alone."

> **Tina English,** Founder and Trustee, Embracing Age

"*Unfailing Love* combines a deep, personal grasp of the experience of dementia with a wonderful sense of what Scripture has to say about it. Powerful stories and reflections bring to life emotional challenges and spiritual questions with which readers will readily identify. These devotions show readers that they are not alone, that lament and questioning are themes of Scripture and that God's promises are true and dependable."

Julia Burton-Jones, Training and Development Lead, Anna Chaplaincy, BRF Ministries

"I wish this book had been available as I watched my mother become so helpless through her aggressive form of Alzheimer's (followed by my father's gentler dementia). It has given me a renewed capacity to engage and empathise with those experiencing dementia, through the range of stories Robin presents. His beautiful simplicity makes this devotional so readable and engaging—a labour of love that will help us love those we care for."

Rev. Dr Jem Hovil, Executive Trustee, BUILD Partners

"These 30 devotions, which draw on real-life stories and experiences from dementia caregivers, have been beautifully written. Many of these reflections have moved me to tears, and I can't recommend *Unfailing Love* highly enough for anyone that supports and cares for a loved one who is suffering with dementia."

Pippa Cramer MBE, Pastoral Care and Seniors Minister, Holy Trinity Church, Claygate

"I've learned in my own mother's Alzheimer's journey that dementia is (as the author of Ecclesiastes described) a crooked line that can't be made straight. If you're exhausted by the failure to problem-solve, wearied by the toll of caregiving, and looking for God in this valley of the shadow of death, take up this book. It will comfort you to remember God carries us as we care."

Jen Pollock Michel, Author, *In Good Time*

Robin Thomson

Unfailing Love

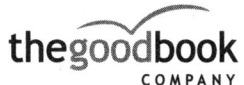

Unfailing Love

© Robin Thomson, 2025

Published by:
The Good Book Company

thegoodbook.com | thegoodbook.co.uk
thegoodbook.com.au | thegoodbook.co.nz

Unless otherwise indicated, Scripture quotations are from The Holy Bible, English Standard Version (ESV), copyright © 2001 by Crossway, a publishing ministry of Good News Publishers. Used by permission. All rights reserved. Emphasis added is the author's own.

All rights reserved. Except as may be permitted by the Copyright Act, no part of this publication may be reproduced in any form or by any means without prior permission from the publisher.

Robin Thomson has asserted his right under the Copyright, Designs and Patents Act 1988 to be identified as author of this work.

Cover design by Drew McCall

ISBN: 9781802543001 | JOB-008067 | Printed in India

Contents

Introduction … 9

Part I: We Have a Heavenly Father Who is Both Loving and Powerful

  1. Knowing God as Father … 14

  2. Knowing God's Character … 17

  3. God's Wise and Fatherly Purpose … 21

  4. The Lord is Good … 25

  5. Receiving from Him Daily … 28

  6. Have You Not Heard? … 33

  7. Lamenting and Believing go Together … 38

Part II: We Are Persons Made in God's Image

  8. Personal Knowledge … 46

  9. Person-Centred Care … 51

  10. I Am Called By Your Name … 56

  11. To Grey Hairs I Will Carry You … 60

  12. Love Wins … 63

Part III: When We Suffer, God Is With Us

    13. How Long?   70

    14. Where Are You, God?   75

    15. Wake Up, God   80

    16. Why Me? Why Not Me?   85

    17. With the Three in the Fiery Furnace   88

    18. Death's Bite Remains   93

Part IV: We Have a Hope Beyond This Life

    19. Going Home   98

    Should We Pray for Healing for Those Living With Dementia?   101

    20. I Shall See Your Face   105

    21. The Weight of Glory   108

    22. Not As She Will Be   113

    Which Person Will We See in the Resurrection Life?   116

Part V: We Are Part of a Loving Community

    23. You Did it to Me   120

    24. Clay Pots   123

25. We Need Friends	126
26. All Things in Common	130
27. When One Member Suffers…	135
28. The Lord Will Keep You	140
29. Love as I Have Loved	145
30. The Last Word	150
Appendix: Responding to Dementia: Helpful Books and Resources	153
Endnotes	167

Introduction

Caring for someone you love through a chronic illness like dementia is a huge privilege but a heavy load too. You do it gladly but find it draining and sometimes overwhelming. You might be facing your experience with courage and hope, or you may have reached a stage where you feel you have little or no respite. You may have good days, but perhaps that is all they are, in the context of long months and years. What does the gospel say to us in this situation?

Here are 30 short reflections on simple gospel truths. At the heart of them all is the assurance of God's unfailing, steadfast love.

But I trust in your unfailing love. (Psalm 13:5, NIV)

God's love is promised to us, and it will never change. We will explore what that means in the context of dementia.

These devotions arise from reflecting on God's word during my own experience when my wife, Shoko, was living with Alzheimer's and I cared for her over a period of nearly seven years. I have written our full story elsewhere,[1] so here I have simply drawn on our experience in some of the reflections, along with the experiences of many others. Shoko died of heart failure in 2018.

How Dementia Affects Us

Dementia has many patterns; there are many kinds of dementia.[2] And our brains are so wonderfully complex that disease affects them in almost infinite ways. Everybody's experience is different, though there are common themes. It's fundamental to remember that people living with dementia are still persons, with abilities, feelings and emotional capacities that persist beyond the limitations in their cognitive or physical ability. A diagnosis of dementia is not the end. There is still much to live for and experience. You will read accounts of joy and opportunity, as well as loss, in the stories here.

In all of this, caregivers—generally family or friends—have a vital place. Caregiving is an amazing role and, for many, a privilege. But it is also demanding, and in a recent survey 54% of caregivers said they were stressed most of the time.[3] None of us would have chosen this role though we carry it out with love and commitment.

It's important to remember that not all those living with dementia need, or want, somebody to care for them. They want to continue being independent and doing what they can for as long as they can. Caring doesn't mean doing everything for the other person. It does mean being available to serve in whatever way is best for them.

These devotions are mostly from the perspective of those who are primary carers for somebody living with dementia. But they are not limited to them. Dementia's effects begin with the person living with dementia but, as when a stone drops into a pool, they ripple out to their family and friends and all their networks. Some talk very openly together about their situation. Others don't or can't. While attitudes are changing in our societies, there is still fear, incomprehension and a preference not to get involved.

Sharing Stories

I am very grateful to those who have shared the stories which you will find interspersed in this book. You may find some of the stories hard to read. All of them come from people whose faith in God is strong and has kept them going. But they have described their situations as they were, sometimes expressing their faith, sometimes simply expressing their pain. They are like the Old Testament psalmists who described their feelings so graphically. Sometimes they saw God's intervention or received his comfort; sometimes not at that time. We agreed not to identify anybody, so all the names have been changed (except for my wife, Shoko).

This book is not intended to replace the many resources that are available for help with dementia (see the appendix for links to a few). My only real advice is to encourage you to build your support network, and perhaps this book may help towards that.

The truths of the gospel that we will look at may well be familiar to you. Believing in these promises gives a sure foundation for our lives. But they will be severely tested through our experiences of caring and of chronic illness. I hope you will find God's strength as you read and reflect on your experience with dementia. You can read these devotions at your own pace and in any order. After each one there are questions for reflection, and you may find it helpful to write your own thoughts in response.

Part I

We Have a Heavenly Father Who Is Both Loving and Powerful

Day 1

Knowing God as Father

When you pray, say: "Father..."

Luke 11:2

Luke's version of the Lord's Prayer begins so simply. To call God "Father" expresses faith in somebody who is connected to us, who cares for us and who has power to intervene in our lives.

In Matthew's Gospel, Jesus taught the same prayer in a different context and added the words "in heaven" (Matthew 6:9), reminding us of the Father's authority. That gives us two sides of the truth about God—he is a loving and dependable Father who is also all-powerful. Whatever happens is under his control, even when we don't understand how. That is a very secure framework for our lives. For me, and perhaps for you too, it's the framework I grew up with, learning it from my parents.

But what happens when that framework is shaken? When

things seem out of control? What if God is all powerful but doesn't love? Or if God is very loving but doesn't really have control?

In the early days of my wife's Alzheimer's, there were times when her behaviour was very strange. She became paranoid about things being stolen and suspicious of people for no good reason (as far as I could see). It led to huge tensions, arguments between us, and embarrassing and painful exchanges with others. At one point the police even became involved.

I didn't understand that this was part of the disease, and I became more and more frustrated, not knowing how to respond. I felt angry and helpless at the same time. I remember days when I literally didn't want to get out of bed in the morning. I was so confused about what was happening to Shoko, and so disturbed.

Often I just lay there and said, "Father". I was putting it all into my heavenly Father's hands. I was saying, "I don't know what to do, but I trust you. You have to help us now."

The Lord's Prayer begins by reminding us of who it is that we are praying to—our Father in heaven. Then we pray that all will acknowledge his greatness ("hallowed be your name"), accept his rule ("Your kingdom come") and fulfil his will ("your will be done"). When we pray like this, we are reminded of who God is, and we align our wills and desires with his will and purpose. The pressures and stress that we are facing fall into a greater perspective.

Some of us may have had a difficult relationship with our own fathers, which makes it harder to understand this kind of relationship with God. In that case, the best place to start is with Jesus' words about the Father as our reference, rather than our own experience. Matthew 6, which contains the Lord's Prayer, is full of references to the Father. He knows all about us, as we see in verses 1, 4, 6 and 18. And this knowledge is not impersonal, like a CCTV camera recording our movements or an algorithm controlling them. It's very personal:

Your Father knows what you need before you ask him.
(v 8)

We don't need to remind him about our needs, but he invites us to speak with him, and he loves to have us ask.

Your heavenly Father knows that you need them all.
(v 32)

He knows that we need food and clothes, and he provides them, just as he feeds the birds and puts flowers in the fields (v 26-33). We can trust him. He is the heavenly Father, who does love me and who is in control.

Reflect

As you face your experience with dementia, what help are you looking for from your heavenly Father? Do you have questions you want to ask him? Or are you just longing for him to do something about your situation?

Write down your needs—remembering that he already knows them. And tell him honestly your current questions, doubts, and pressures.

Then say, "Father".

Day 2

Knowing God's Character

The name of the LORD is a strong tower; the righteous man runs into it and is safe.

Proverbs 18:10

Mary's Story

My husband, Graham, was diagnosed with Alzheimer's disease in 2009 when he was 75. He had enjoyed a fulfilling career as a doctor in mission work in Asia and in the UK. He had retired as a surgeon and GP but continued to work with two charitable trusts which he had helped to set up. He was very fit, enjoying tennis and any physical activity, and had many responsibilities in our church as well. It was a full and active life. We saw all this eroded in the years that followed.

Graham had to withdraw from so many parts of his life. He was aware of what was happening to him, because of his medical background, so he knew that he had to hand things over. But he didn't realise how much the loss would affect him. He felt diminished, with a sense that he was losing his identity, as he forgot who people were and it became harder for people to keep on talking to him.

Graham talked openly about what was happening, but even he didn't really appreciate how it would develop. He read a lot of information about dementia at the beginning, but it didn't help him practically. If anything, it made him more depressed.

I was in a similar situation: I knew a lot from my background as a medical social worker, but when it came to the practical daily reality, I felt quite impotent. It was hard to come to terms with such loss.

Mary's feelings echo the experience of so many. Dementia brings loss. Author Wendy Mitchell, who wrote her own story of grappling with dementia, called herself "somebody I used to know".[4] And receiving a diagnosis of dementia can be just as devastating for the caregiver as for the one given the diagnosis. What happens next? Is this the end of our life as we have known it? Where do we get reliable information and advice?

Where do you turn in the face of such uncertainty or loss? Proverbs 18:10 suggests that "the name of the Lord" can become a place of safety. What does that mean? Psalm 9:9-10 says something similar: the Lord is "a stronghold in times of trouble", and it adds, "Those who know your name put their trust in you".

The name of the Lord is mentioned both times. God's name reflects who he is. Knowing his name means knowing his character. When we consider the many names of God in the Bible, we can begin to understand his nature.

Look at David's description of God at the beginning of Psalm 18:

I love you, O Lord, my strength.
The Lord is my rock and my fortress and my deliverer,
  my God, my rock, in whom I take refuge. (v 1-2)

The names that God is called here (strength, fortress, deliverer, rock) reflect David's confidence in and gratitude to the one who had "rescued him from the hand of all his enemies, and from the hand of Saul", as the opening of the psalm describes.

Turning to a different Old Testament figure, the prophet Nahum, in the face of devastating oppression from the Assyrian Empire, repeats the picture of the Lord as "a stronghold in the day of trouble". And he adds, "The Lord is good … he knows those who take refuge in him" (Nahum 1:7).

It's not just that we know his character: that "the Lord is good". He also knows us; he knows what we are experiencing, what we need and what our limits are.

Mary found her loss hard and painful. But she was able to persevere because she knew God's character. She and her husband had both experienced God's faithfulness, guidance and care over many years. She was able to remember this and turn once more to God for strength and security as she and Graham faced this new and very dark challenge. Later she was able to share some of what she had learned with others facing the same kind of loss. She brought hope and strength to them too, through setting up the kind of support group that she would have welcomed herself.

Knowing God's character—knowing that he understands us and our situation—makes us realise that we are safe in his will. Coming to him reminds us that we are in his strong tower—and in that place we have security and hope, whatever is going on around us.

"You, O Lord, have not forsaken those who seek you" continues Psalm 9:10. We seek him and find safety in him.

Reflect

What have you experienced of God's character? Which names of God are more meaningful for you? Write them down and consider what they reveal about your Father's provision for you today.

Day 3

God's Wise and Fatherly Purpose

I have learned in whatever state I am in to be content ... I can do all things through him who strengthens me.

Philippians 4:11, 13

Rebecca's Story

On the whole, we are doing okay, but I am coming to terms with what I have lost because of my husband's Alzheimer's:

- *No more holidays because new information overload is detrimental to his wellbeing.*

- *No more eating out (saving me having to cook a meal)—he no longer wants to do that.*

- *No more days out because he would get anxious if I was gone for too long.*

- *No guaranteed uninterrupted time when I sit down to do something, as I never know when he might need me.*

It's hard to stay content when a person you love is changing before your eyes and your family feels bereaved already. It's hard to go on caring unselfishly when you are so tired. Where does your contentment come from?

Contentment may be the single most absent quality from our lives today, both as individuals and as a society. Our whole economy is based on consumer confidence and spending. It needs us to keep wanting—and spending—more. And in our individual lives there are so many areas where we wrestle with discontentment, not least when we experience the illness of loved ones.

Sheila describes her challenges as a caregiver for her mother:

It's her utter dependence on us, now all the time, that becomes very tiring. It means structuring her day, finding activities, helping her eat and walk because she has lost much of her mobility. Then tackling her fear of the dark when evening comes. And just her boredom too. We want to enable her to stay at home, so that means managing the carers. We do our best to keep her engaged in community life—and our church is a vital link in this. But there is such an impact on the rest of life that we are juggling all the time.

In the context of today's verse, Paul was writing from prison in Rome—perhaps on death row and certainly facing that possibility—yet he could say that he was contented, whatever the situation. Contentment is an attitude of "submitting to and delighting in God's wise and fatherly disposal [i.e. his arrangement of our situation] in any condition," John McArthur says in his commentary on this passage. It comes "only from being rightly related to God and trusting in his sovereign, loving, purposeful providence".[5]

Another person who was imprisoned, like Paul, for his faith in Jesus was Lewis de Marolles. Living in France in the 1680s, he suffered inhumane treatment for many years: kept in chains, moved from dungeon to dungeon, and forced to serve as a galley slave. His captors constantly tried to crush his confidence in God and his hope of eternal life. But Marolles continued to call God his "dear and true friend". He wrote, "I am persuaded that all states and conditions in which it shall please him to put me are those states in which he judges I shall glorify him better than in an infinite number of others which he might allot me."[6]

Can we really believe that for ourselves? Am I content with what God has given me in my life? Is this really the situation in which I can best glorify God?

Accepting this feels painful, but there's also something reassuring in it. When we are weak, we turn to the one "who strengthens [us]" (Philippians 4:13). His power is displayed most clearly in our weakness (2 Corinthians 12:9). We remember again that our heavenly Father knows our situation better than we do. He knows that this is the place in which we can best glorify him. He has chosen it for us; it's not an accident. That doesn't mean that he wishes sickness or disaster or unhappy events. But he allows us to experience them in this fallen world. And he knows that as we accept them from his hand and trust his "wise and fatherly" purpose, it will enable us—and others—to see more of his good character.

In the centre of the circle
Of the love of God I stand.
Here there are no second causes;
All must come from his dear hand.[7]

Reflect

What are the challenges to contentment in your situation? Are you, like Sheila, juggling all the time? What are the things that most irritate or trouble you?

Tell them to your Father and ask that you would find contentment in him alone.

Day 4

The Lord Is Good

*The LORD is good; his steadfast love endures for
ever, and his faithfulness to all generations.*

Psalm 100:5

When Santosh's father had a stroke, it changed the condition of his dementia. From being able to continue quietly and peacefully each day, his actions became erratic and difficult to manage. His doctor was a good friend, who also ran a small care home. He offered a place for Santosh's father where he could be cared for in security. It seemed the right place for him, but Santosh and his wife, Miriam, remembered it as "the hardest decision of our lives. We cried for three days as we tried to make up our minds." In the end, they trusted their friend, and they trusted God, believing that he had provided this solution for them.

Psalm 100 assures us that we can trust God. It is bold and exuberant as it invites us to praise God with singing.

We may not always feel like making a "joyful noise unto the Lord" (v 1, KJV), but behind the loud affirmation is the quiet assurance that we belong to God (v 3) and that he is good (v 5). His attitude toward us is "steadfast love". This is the Hebrew word *hesed*, which is also translated as "unfailing love" (NLT), "loving and kind" (TLB), and "mercy" (KJV).

Hesed is connected to God's covenant with his people, when he freed them from Egypt (Exodus 34:6). When Jonathan makes a covenant with David (1 Samuel 20:14-17) he asks him to go on showing *hesed* (steadfast love, loyalty) as the Lord has shown it. Because it is based on God's covenant relationship, this is promise love, committed love. God our Father has committed himself to us, so his love never changes; it "endures for ever".

It isn't always easy to hold on to that. Is God's love enduring for Vera, who is unable to move from her bed or chair? And for Paul, as he cares for her? Hazel has Parkinson's and her brilliant scholar husband, Martin, has just been diagnosed with dementia. Is this God's goodness to them? Many others have faced agonising decisions about how to care for parents or family members, like Santosh and Miriam.

How do we reconcile this with God's goodness? Is there room to doubt? God's people have raised those questions plenty of times, and we will explore them again later. But even as the Bible writers ask questions, especially in the Psalms, they hold on to the framework of belief in God, the Creator who "made us" (Psalm 100:3). We belong to him as his people, and he provides for us as "the sheep of his pasture".

Without this belief, our lives are uncertain. We may still have the love of family and friends or other relationships that help to sustain us. But even deeper is the unfailing love of the Creator: the Father who doesn't change.

Howard and Sue are in their late eighties and now live in sheltered accommodation. Sue has been living with Alzheimer's for over seven years, and Howard cares for her. They have managed so far—not without ups and downs. They are very different: she has always been independent and loves to talk; Howard prefers reading or sitting at his desk.

"We have a row every day," says Howard.

"But with a small 'r'," Sue replies.

The "row" is usually over time, or cooking and shopping. Despite her extrovert temperament, Sue has had times of great discouragement: "Nobody wants me these days; I'm always wrong". What has kept them both going, through all the turbulence and adjustments, is their settled faith, cultivated over a lifetime, with a pattern of prayer, reading their Bibles and joining with others for fellowship. Sue's conclusion: "I just think that the Lord has been very good to us, really".

His enduring love will sustain, to the very end of our lives and in the life to come.

Reflect

In what ways have you experienced God's steadfast love (his unfailing promise love)? Can you think of promises that you have received, as you have listened to and studied his word? How does that strengthen your faith in his goodness?

Day 5

Receiving from Him Daily

Therefore do not be anxious about tomorrow, for tomorrow will be anxious for itself. Let the day's own trouble be sufficient for the day.

Matthew 6:34 (RSV)

"Normally we would be out and about," a friend wrote to me, as his wife faced increasing physical limitations. I wondered what he meant by "normally"—the old days that would never come back?

"Julie would be less aware of her limitations because there would be plenty to see and people to interact with. Please pray for the wisdom to find things that are uplifting to occupy her each day."

Another friend, facing his own increasing limitations from Parkinson's disease, wrote, "It's hard to take Jesus' words seriously and not to worry about tomorrow."

I understood what they both meant. "This is going to

be a long haul," I wrote in my journal, a few months after Shoko had declined into her new normal pattern of life, in which nothing was quite the same as before and everyday life was confused. How long would it continue like that? There was no way of knowing.

We couldn't plan our lives in the way we used to. She was losing her abilities, and as a result I could no longer do the things that I would like to. Each day brought the same challenge: how to help her occupy the day with meaningful and enjoyable activities.

Can we take Jesus' words seriously? He said to his disciples, "Therefore do not be anxious about tomorrow…" There are many things that all of us need, and as we have seen, Jesus promises that "your heavenly Father knows that you need them all". He is aware of the cost of living, he is aware of the challenges of dementia, and he will supply all that you need (Matthew 6:32-33).

But he does it one day at a time.

Jesus' words reminded me of the widow who looked after Elijah in a time of famine (1 Kings 17:8-16). Elijah asked her to use the last of her flour and oil to feed him. In return, he promised that her jar of flour and bottle of oil would last miraculously until the famine was over. And they did: "The jar of flour was not spent, neither did the jug of oil become empty, according to the word of the Lord that he spoke by Elijah" (v 16). This widow had great faith. But when I thought more about it, I realised that it wasn't a one-off act of belief. God didn't fill a huge storehouse with everything she needed for the duration of the drought. She would have had to go to her meagre storeroom each day, look at the "handful" (v 12) of flour in the jar and the "little" oil in the bottle, and believe that there would be enough—just for that day.

When God supplied the Israelites in the desert with manna, they collected it each day, and there was just the right amount—not too much, not too little (Exodus 16:21). As I reflected on these stories, I began to pray each day that "today I will be able to love, serve and care for Shoko in the best way for her". I asked our friends to pray this for us too.

A friend recently wrote to me after receiving his diagnosis, "Last night I felt strongly that God was telling me to trust him for the future, and to enjoy the present. I feel much relieved with this message." It doesn't mean that we don't need to think ahead or plan. But Jesus was right. As we receive each day from God, he gives what we need for that day—no more, no less.

Reflect

How much flour and oil or manna do you need today? Tell God your particular needs at this time; then ask him for the faith and strength to trust him to provide for them today. Turn that into a prayer that you can repeat each day.

Rachel's Story

In 2008 I began to notice that my mother wasn't quite right. It was just one tiny step at a time, so it took quite a while to realise this—especially because she covered it up.

Once, she had bought a spool of string for her garden, having forgotten that she had just purchased the same thing a few days earlier. As I walked in, she was staring at both spools, completely puzzled. She looked at me and said, "Oh, Rachel, I think I bought this one for you".

Another time, she invited me for a meal. When I turned up, she had remembered the date and done all the shopping with the right ingredients. She told me to go and sit with my father while she prepared the meal. After a while, I went to the kitchen and found her distressed because she couldn't cope; she couldn't organise things or remember the sequence of what to do when.

It was a slow deterioration from then on. We had live-in carers as my father was also ill. He died a couple of years after her diagnosis. The doctor told us that she needed a routine: everything should be the same—the plates and cutlery and so on. We should let her do whatever she wanted—just help to facilitate her—and she would be peaceful and contented. That was true: she mostly wanted to watch films on TV or cut up pieces of tissue into little squares and pile them up. But as soon as there was any difference or new people came to the house, she would become highly agitated.

She knew all of her family; she knew we were special people to her, and she never forgot us when we saw her. But she didn't understand that we were her children. Sometimes I would drive home crying after a visit, but because I saw her frequently, I came to terms with it earlier. But it was difficult for my siblings to come for brief visits and see our mother like that. When somebody has dementia, you have to accept that that is who they are now. You don't always know how to handle it, and you have to figure it out yourself.

I learned a lot from the carers. They just picked up all the unique things about my mum and cared for her in a way that suited who she was. I found that my experience as a teacher with small children helped me because I had learned to use talking to soothe. On so many occasions, I felt God prompting me in certain ways during this time. He really does help you when you are up against it.

Day 6

Have You Not Heard?

*Have you not known? Have you not heard? The
LORD is the everlasting God, the Creator of the ends
of the earth. He does not faint or grow weary.*

Isaiah 40:28

"I'm feeling so tired and puzzled at what is happening to us."

"Sometimes I feel God is remote and uncaring. And even if he cares, I have no energy to respond. It's all very confusing."

God's Old Testament people, Israel, had similar feelings as they were cast off into exile in Babylon. They were in deep trouble, under a powerful conqueror, spiritually oppressed, with no vision for the future.

The prophet Isaiah brought them a vision of God, the all-powerful Creator, coming to his people. It is a compelling vision. "Comfort, comfort my people" are the opening words of chapter 40, familiar perhaps from

Handel's *Messiah*. "Behold your God!" says Isaiah (v 9). Our God "comes with might" (v 10), but he gently cares for his flock—the lambs and their mothers (v 11). He is the almighty Creator (v 12-24); the heavens and the earth and everybody in them are "as nothing before him" (v 17).

"To whom then will you compare me?" he asks (v 25). The stars are all his creation, known to him by name (v 26). These stars are not powerful gods, as the Babylonians believed at that time, nor cold, glittering objects of measureless space, as people think today. They are his army, lined up according to his orders:

> *[He] leads them out like an army, he knows how many there are and calls each one by name! (v 26, GNT)*

It's good to look away from ourselves, remembering God's power in ordering all things in the world, both large and small. Hear his words of assurance; he is "the everlasting God, the Creator of the ends of the earth. He does not faint or grow weary" (v 28).

We, however, certainly become weary.

Dr John Dunlop is a geriatric physician who also cared for both his own parents when they had Alzheimer's. So the book he wrote about dementia has medical authority but is also compassionate and honest, with insight from both outside and inside his own experience.[8] His chapter on the challenges for caregivers lists the possible demands—physical, mental, social, emotional and spiritual. As I read it, I ticked them off and thought, "He understands our situation".

Some of the demands can be distressing; some are just minor irritations. The rows may have only a small "r"—by themselves, they may not matter very much. But cumulatively the effect is draining. Everybody's situation is different, but for many the word that sums it up is "relentless".

When we feel discouraged or confused (and it's *when*, not *if* with dementia), it is encouraging to remember God's measureless power and energy. But we may still think, "How does that help me in my weariness? I have no strength these days."

Isaiah's next verse tells us:

He gives power to the faint,
and to him who has no might
he increases strength. (v 29)

These are words to take hold of—a promise to claim. He promises to give us strength, as we "wait for the Lord" (v 31). When we feel we don't have energy even to do that, it might be that others can help us through conversations or the words of songs, or when we join with them as we meet in church.

In your weariness, remember your Creator God, who never grows tired of caring for you.

Reflect

When you feel exhausted, frustrated or confused, what helps you to remember God's strength? Reflect on Isaiah's description of God in chapter 40. What kind of attitude do we need in order to "wait for the Lord"? Can you ask for others' help in this?

Anne's Story

"I should like to meet your mother! Is she still alive?" my mother asked me one day.

She hadn't recognised me as her daughter for several years, but I mostly felt that she knew there was some kind of connection—a college friend, she'd guess. She'd look blankly across the breakfast table when Dad would say, "She's your dawh-ter!... and I'm your huzz-band!"

His orator finger would obligingly prod the air to remind himself that this was all theatrical stuff and the show had to go on, however tired we all were of playing the parts assigned to us by our new director: dementia.

"It doesn't matter, Dad," I'd say. And it didn't for me. I was there to give Dad a break. I'd try to stay for about a week every couple of months—Scotland to southwest England was not a simple journey. Two of my siblings lived close by and visited frequently, sorting out issues as they arose. I felt I could help with the long stretch of each day and relieve some of the exhaustion he felt, come evening, when Mum was not for heading bed-wards. It's always surprising just how many additional jobs and challenges dementia slips under the front door each day.

It didn't matter to Mum either, as her early childhood faith had fixed her feet firmly onto a bedrock of security and happiness. But it did matter to my dad. He was responsible for her safety and her care. He had risen to the challenges of managing all the shopping and cooking and "unmuddling" of the house so late in life—and he did it with flair! But he had his own mobility limitations and a stroke had made speech a challenge, especially when tired. However, he wasn't going to let dementia wipe out all trace of his long and happy marriage.

So, when Mum hardly touched her breakfast one morning and went back to bed, I took her coffee in to her and sat on her bed.

"Are you okay, Mum? How are you feeling?" She didn't answer but looked blankly at me.

"You didn't eat much breakfast; do you feel sick?" Silence.

"Is your head sore? Your tummy? Is it your knee again?" She looked surprised and then blank again.

"You okay, Mum?"

I then remembered to replace my look of concern with a big smile.

She smiled back and said, "Thank you. I'll just wait,"

"Good idea, Mum! You look nice and comfy here. I'll come back in a little bit."

Day 7

Lamenting and Believing Go Together

*I kept my faith, even when I said,
"I am greatly afflicted."*

Psalm 116:10, NRSV

When you've had times of feeling discouraged, have you found yourself complaining in your heart? And if so, did you feel bad about it? *Surely I should be coping better than this... Have I lost my faith?*

One Sunday morning, Shoko and I were in church as usual. It was good to be there, but I felt quite down. It wasn't (only) self-pity; I really was finding things difficult. We sang a familiar hymn which spoke about "living water", which included these beautiful lines:

*Who can faint while such a river
Ever flows their thirst to assuage?*[9]

I was immediately challenged. Why was I feeling "faint"? I should be doing better; where was my faith? Feeling guilty, I resolved that I had better talk about it with our vicar at our next regular chat—my conversations with him had been so helpful to me.

But in the next few days, I received an email from a Christian leader in Sri Lanka, describing how he often walked beside the river near his house, pouring out his heart's concerns and crying out to God—over personal issues, difficulties in the church, the struggles and pain of Sri Lanka at that time. He quoted these words from Psalm 116:10: "I kept my faith, even when I said, 'I am greatly afflicted'."

"Lament and faith can exist together," he said. The psalmist had cried out to God, but he continued to believe. So, the leader commented, when we cry out to God, it doesn't mean that we don't trust him or that our faith is failing. In fact, the opposite is true: crying out to God can be a sign of our faith. Lamenting and believing go together.

Over a third of the book of Psalms consists of "psalms of lament". Individuals or whole communities are bringing their sorrow and their needs to God. Some of these psalms are really anguished cries. We will look at a few of them later on.

My Sri Lankan friend didn't know my situation, but his words were exactly what I needed to hear. Crying out to God didn't mean that I had lost my faith. It was *OK to be Not OK,* as the title of a recent book on the psalms of lament puts it.[10] Of course it was easy and understandable to feel self-pity, but I found there was a fine line between a genuine expression of pain and self-centred pity. I had to remember to "[keep] my faith" and bring all that I was feeling to God, as the psalm writers do.

Lamenting doesn't mean that we don't believe. The psalms encourage us to acknowledge our pain and disappointments and bring them to God; he listens to all our cries.

Reflect

When you feel sadness and pain, do you feel that you are just complaining? Do you feel guilty about it? Can you bring your feelings directly to God so that your lament and your belief go together?

David and Emily's Story

David was in his mid-fifties when he was diagnosed with Parkinson's, which then developed to include Parkinson's-related dementia.

What were the first effects?

David: I was constantly tired and anxious, and my speech was affected. Sometimes it was extremely difficult to get out the words I was thinking of. Now I have developed symptoms of Parkinson's-related dementia. Half the time I am completely normal, and I understand everything. The other half of the time I have hallucinations or forget things or "freeze" as though I am asleep. I find these times of confusion very hard. And it is very difficult for my wife.

You have spent over 30 years studying the brain, so you know exactly what is going on. How do you cope with it on a daily basis?

David: I have felt frustrated, not being able to do things that I want to do—many of them very worthy things. I think I can do things as before, but it can take so long that I never even begin. It's difficult not to be in control, so I can get depressed and anxious. For example, I worry about the future. Emily, who cares for me, might die. Or I might die, and then who would look after her? Sometimes I worry about my "absences"—that I might not come out of them but just continue in that state.

Emily: It's hard to keep up with the constantly changing medication. We have to keep on making huge adjustments as we determine where to focus David's increasingly limited energies. Each time there is a slide down, we learn to adjust and develop new ways of thinking. These days, we have all kinds of things that we would never have thought of a year ago, like his special chair and wheelchair, or handgrips around the house.

Did you ever think that David would get better?

Emily: We read a verse in the Bible that promised, "Don't be afraid ... I have called you by name ... when you pass through the waters, I will be with you" (Isaiah 43:1-2, ICB). I interpreted this to mean that David would not be healed but that God would be with us through all his illness.

David: I was sure that I would recover because I had always got round any obstacle in the past.

Does faith become more difficult as we get older or more frail?

David: Yes. Sometimes I feel my relationship with God is more distant. I realise that I used to rely on my own ability to solve problems. Now I don't have the same abilities, but I haven't yet replaced them with genuine trust in God. In the past I used to get by with half-faith. I didn't need to trust God fully; there was always a way out of difficulties. Now I need to get to know God better, or life would be miserable. When I used to talk to others who felt that way, I would counsel them that they are made by God and he does not make rubbish. But I found it difficult to apply that to myself. It takes a long time for God to change us so that we learn to trust him and not rely on ourselves. I sometimes wonder what my ministry is these days; I used to be so active in many areas.

Emily: You may not be so active now, but who you are in Christ is definitely visible. Your humble attitude is the fruit of many years of humbling yourself before God.

Part II

We Are Persons Made in God's Image

Day 8

Personal Knowledge

O Lord, you have searched me and known me!
You know when I sit down and when I rise up ...
Even before a word is on my tongue ...
you know it altogether.

Psalm 139:1-4

David, the writer of this psalm, sees his whole life laid out before God. Every detail, every moment, is known to him. Nothing happens without God's knowledge, his care, his plan. No wonder that David says:

Such knowledge is too wonderful for me;
it is high; I cannot attain it. (v 6)

The thought that God knows us so intimately and cares in such detail is truly wonderful. But can it really be true when we face a diagnosis like dementia? Did God really plan for the people we love to become so different?

"I feel sad that my mother isn't as she used to be," our daughter said when Shoko began to change. *Is this the same person?* we asked.

"Alzheimer's is so cruel," a friend said one day. "It makes your loved one disappear."

"We are managing okay," another friend told me. "But I just want my husband to be like he was before." We wanted the same for Shoko, but we knew it wouldn't happen.

Around this time we were lent a book: *I'm Still Here* by John Zeisel.[11] He pointed out that the person with Alzheimer's is still a person with whom we can relate, though it is a different relationship. It's the same person, but it's also not the same person. We need to comprehend this change because we can't go back to the old relationship. But we can build a new relationship.

Reading Zeisel made so much sense of things that had puzzled us, but it was hard; we were sad to let go of things that we had treasured in Shoko's personality. There was also joy, however, in finding new ways to relate to her.

Although Shoko could still respond with love and affection, we wondered about others whose dementia really did seem to make them "disappear". Vera, a friend who had been very kind to Shoko in her illness, was now herself unable to speak. She had declined rapidly and could only sit in her chair all day. Had the person who she was really gone?

For many, these are agonising questions. What value does a person have when they have lost all means of relating to others? Some would argue, not much. "The real person has gone already and all that's left is just the body," said the philosopher Mary Warnock.[12] We may not express it so starkly, but we can feel bewildered when it seems we are losing the people that we knew: "It matters that they no longer remember or communicate with us. It matters that we feel we are losing them in fundamental ways."[13]

Is there any point? Is anybody still there?

Even at a human level, there are good reasons to answer yes and to continue to relate to them in love. The real self is still there; it takes love to find it.[14] One time when I visited Vera and Paul, she was listening to gospel songs that he had found for her, with simple words and appealing tunes. She was alert and communicated, without words, her pleasure at seeing me. Paul's loving care was sustaining her real self, even when others could not see it.

From God's perspective the answer is clear, as the writer David knows:

All the stages of my life were spread out before you ...
before I'd even lived one day. (v 16, MSG)

God knew us in the womb when we could not speak and had no knowable personality. We are still persons, whom he knows intimately and cares for, even if we lose our speech or other abilities. He holds us in his infinite knowledge all through our lives.

So, the form of our love may change but we go on loving, just as our heavenly Father does.

Reflect

How have you found ways to develop a new kind of relationship as you grapple with the effects of dementia on you and the person you love? How does God's personal knowledge of both of you help you in doing that?

Sushila's Story

Sometimes when Ritu wakes, she will flash a smile, or there will be a flicker of recognition when somebody speaks, but that is now very infrequent. To the outsider it seems that she makes no response at all. But the family keep talking to her. Every day there are several FaceTime calls from family members around the world. With the screen in front of her, she can see who is calling and they can see her. Her sister now speaks to her in Gujarati, the language they spoke in their childhood, and calls her by the name she used as a girl. That brings more reaction—though now even that doesn't work very often.

Despite the apparent lack of response, our family go on treating her as a valued person. They try to give her food that she likes and keep speaking to her every day. I do my best to stimulate her—perhaps teasing her or her husband.

Jessica's Story

My grandmother was born in 1911 in South Africa. She was a wonderful homemaker. She cooked superbly, loved gardening, adored having family and friends round, was a skilled dressmaker and did beautiful smocking. She loved games, and our childhood visits often involved hockey with walking sticks in the garden and lots of concerts.

Why am I telling you this? Because, when we meet someone with dementia, it is so easy to get stuck in the present sadness that we can ignore all the loves and skills and past experiences of that person. The muddle and confusion can dominate, or the silence can put us off sitting for any length with that person. But that person is known and loved by God, created in his image and with a purpose.

My grandmother started showing signs of confusion and memory loss a year or so after my grandfather died suddenly. She was 76 then. She carried on living by herself for two more years, but she started barricading herself in and fear at night became an issue. My parents moved her to a semi-sheltered flat, within walking distance of us, and she started needing more attention and care. I would visit her every day after teaching, and the conversations soon became predictable and repetitive. Sometimes I would cut my visit short as I just felt too tired to cope with the conversation, and then I would feel guilty that I had failed to make that visit special. Other times, I played Scrabble or read the Bible to her, giving her truths to hold on to.

Day 9

Person-Centred Care

But Zion said, "The LORD has forsaken me;
my Lord has forgotten me."
... Yet I will not forget you.
Behold, I have engraved you on the palms of my hands.

Isaiah 49:14-16

Painting hands with henna is common across the Middle East and the Indian subcontinent, especially for brides. The beautiful patterns can stay for several days, but eventually wear off. But in this passage, God's hands are marked indelibly. And the image engraved there is of us, his people. He can never forget us.

Psalm 139 spoke of God's intimate knowledge of us—here we see it is also his permanent knowledge of us. Both passages assure us that God always sees us as persons he has made in his image (Genesis 1:27); he has redeemed us, and we belong to him (Isaiah 43:1).

So we hold on to our belief that people who appear to have lost much of their personality are still persons whom God can never forget. We can express that truth when we, God's people, continue to remember and relate to them.

Thirty years ago, Dr Tom Kitwood re-emphasised the concept of person-centred care for those living with dementia. He found that dementia doesn't progress in a linear fashion, and it varies from person to person. One of the most important factors in this is the quality of care and relationships. It is in relationship that a person's sense of self remains.[15] We are nourished and affirmed by our personal connections with others. For all of us, they help to give us our sense of worth and much more besides.

Kitwood researched what people with dementia need. He found that it began with love at the centre, expressed in five ways, like a flower's petals. These are: *comfort* or warmth, *attachment, being included* and *occupied,* and *having an identity.* It is this kind of care that affirms the person; and it entails recognition, respect and trust.[16]

We are all dependent on God and on each other. We just become more aware of this when we see the effects of dementia, and we have a vital role to care for those affected, just as the Bible emphasises the importance of caring for the poor, vulnerable, widows and orphans. This is what God sees as "pure and undefiled" religion (James 1:27).

Caregivers are the "keepers of dignity and personhood" for those living with dementia.[17] We not only care for them in our human capacity as those who love them; we actually represent God's deeper love and indelible memory. He cannot and will not let them go: they are engraved on his palms.

Knowing this, we continue relating to them in love. The many practical ways in which we do this are all expressions of God's unfailing love. And a small action can have a great effect, as a chaplain working for Anna Chaplaincy[18] recalls:

In my local dementia care home, Margaret, who had recently arrived, was finding it hard to settle. She was reluctant to leave her room or join in any activities. I had asked the children at my church if they would like to write a "card of kindness" to a nominated resident at the home. Margaret was so delighted with her card, from a little girl called Polly, that she wrote back to her, making a little parcel with some rose petals and a pencil. She was told that I was coming to visit with our gospel choir that evening, and if she brought it there, I would take it and deliver it for her. So Margaret left her room and came to the concert to give me the parcel. She was then moved to tears by the gospel songs. She started singing along and clapping with everyone else. Since then, she joins in everything!

Polly's card told Margaret that God had not forgotten her.

Reflect

What ways have you found to communicate love, in all its different aspects, and to maintain relationship? Think about those five petals—comfort, attachment, being included, being occupied, and having an identity. What actions could you take to express each one of them?

Anne's Story

Mum increasingly loved soft toys, to my dad's embarrassment. She would hold them and position them over the side of her chair, so that they could comment on life. "He's a little bored today", or "He's sniffing the air outside". Then I could have nice conversations with Paddington (made by her own mother—a real vintage character), or the soft-furred white lamb (with the sideways smile that Mum cherished), and we could explore all kinds of ideas and thoughts without having to think very hard. We both had fun, punning and being silly, while Dad retreated into the comfort of a television programme or a pre-recorded Proms concert. Mum had stopped being able to enjoy these, as the screen made it look as if the televised people were in the room with us, and it would be rude to ask them to leave. Paddington understood and distracted her with little games and wise words about what was going on.

Of course, there were many occasions when Mum did not feel at ease, and we could sense the distortion of memories jostling for space in her head, especially when things were happening around her. I might have felt that I was doing my best to reassure her, but in fact reassurance often came from within herself. She once told my daughter, "I find that if I'm frightened, I just sing, and it makes it better". Different songs surfaced at different times, but a frequent one was a variation on "Absolutely gentle, infinitely near, this is God our Father; what have we to fear?" Another time my daughter asked, "Are you okay, Granny?" when she was sitting with her eyes closed. The reply came: "I'm just counting my blessings!"

Mum's graciousness did stem from her trust in God, but that was an ongoing act of will on her part, and she held on to him right through the most challenging times. A lifetime of learning and repeating Christian songs proved to be the best training for living with her dementia.

Day 10

I Am Called by Your Name

*I am called by your name, O LORD, God of hosts
… I sat alone because your hand was upon me.*

Jeremiah 15:16-17

Jeremiah experienced God's intimate, personal knowledge of him. God had told him, "Before I formed you in the womb I knew you" (Jeremiah 1:5). That must have been a huge assurance. But despite this, Jeremiah was tempted to despair, as the people did not listen to his message for over 40 years. God's call on his life separated him from others. He felt alone.

Jeremiah felt cut off, not only from other people, but also from God. If God betrayed him too, that would be the end. "Why is my pain unceasing … Will you be to me like a deceitful brook, like waters that fail?" he asks (15:18).

People living with dementia can feel the same. Robert Davis, a Baptist pastor diagnosed with Alzheimer's, found his faith faltering. He could not read the Bible nor pray as he wanted. He was "grasping for the peace of the Saviour ... but finding nothing ... I concluded that the only reason for such darkness must be spiritual ... I could only lie there and cry, 'O God, why? Why?'"[19]

When Jeremiah cried out in the same way, the Lord repeated the promise he had made at his first calling, years before: "They shall not prevail over you, for I am with you" (15:20; compare 1:19). The Lord had not forgotten Jeremiah. Jesus repeated this same promise to his disciples as he commissioned them: "I am with you always". He is truly Immanuel, God with us—always (Matthew 28:20; 1:23).

We may feel "the loneliness of dementia",[20] which can affect those living with dementia and those close to them. Just as he was with Jeremiah, God is with us. He is with us through his people, as we relate in love to each other, but more than that, he is with us directly through his Holy Spirit. As people made by God, we are held in his memory. So he does not let us go, even when those we love may appear to have forgotten everything—including God.[21]

Christine Bryden, living with dementia, believes:

I might have difficulty feeling the presence of God or being able to speak the words of a prayer in my mind, but I can commune without words. As my cognition fades, my spirituality can flourish as an important source of identity ... I can seek an identity by simply being me, a person created in the image of God.[22]

When we pray, even at the best of times, we "do not know what to pray for as we ought". But always, "the Spirit helps us in our weakness ... the Spirit himself intercedes for us with groanings too deep for words" (Romans 8:26). How much more true and relevant for the one whose mental grasp may be slipping and who has weakened in other ways.

God communes with our loved ones through his Spirit. He knows their innermost thoughts and feelings:

He who searches the hearts of humans knows what is the mind of the Spirit, because the Spirit intercedes for the saints according to the will of God. (v 27)

And as God understands both our deepest longings and the longings of those we care for, even when we and they may not be able to articulate them, he wills perfectly what is best for us. Whatever our cognitive state, his Spirit is always with us.

Reflect

Have you experienced the loneliness of dementia? How have you found that God has communicated that he is with you—either directly or through others? What steps could you take to keep on reminding yourself of the presence of the Holy Spirit within you?

Sarah's Story

We may sometimes be surprised by people's sense of loving God and being loved by him whilst living with dementia, as an Anna Chaplain discovered.

At one of the Vintage Messy Church sessions I lead in the care home, we helped the residents decorate little mirrors with stick-on flowers and butterflies, and we used peel-off letters to write their names and "God loves me" across the top.

One lady, Janet, always appeared quite lost in her dementia, so I sat and helped her. As we looked at the completed mirror, I said to her, "Janet, do you know how much God loves you?" And she instantly replied with such a beaming smile, "Oh yes, I do, and I love him right back every day!"

The next week she had completely forgotten the mirror. But when I prayed with her, she said again, "I love God always in my heart".

Anne's Story

I began to realise, as I tried to help my mother, that I needed to relax. Mum loved the verse, "My grace is sufficient for you" (2 Corinthians 12:9). That was a kindlier concept to keep in mind than the verse that kept popping into my head when several challenges came at once: "Sufficient unto the day is the evil thereof" (Matthew 6:34, KJV). My verse helped me clean up, and Mum's verse helped us relax and be thankful!

Day 11

To Grey Hairs I Will Carry You

Listen to me, O house of Jacob ...
who have been borne by me from before your birth,
carried from the womb;
even to your old age I am he,
and to grey hairs I will carry you.
I have made, and I will bear;
I will carry and will save.

Isaiah 46:3-4

What happens as we get older? Who will care for us? It's a question for us all, but especially for those affected by dementia. What happens if my partner can't carry on? How can our children cope alongside their own family challenges? What if there is nobody to support us?

Anthony wonders how he will care for his wife, as he is not well himself. Their daughter has her career ahead of her, and he feels it's unfair to depend on her. Thinking about their future makes Anthony feel a "terrible crippling anxiety and sleeplessness about so many things. I cannot sleep after 4 a.m., and I then suffer dizzying periods of weakness every day as a result."

"Prepare for every eventuality," my friend Brian advised. "Perhaps you should consider a care home or a live-in carer? Explore all the options. When the time comes, you will know what to do." His own parents had become concerned for their old age. They had spent many years serving in Africa. Now they needed care for themselves and looked for a live-in carer. The first person whom the agency sent to them was from the same African country where they had lived. They understood each other's culture and ways. They were amazed at God's care for them in their old age and weakness.

But perhaps this isn't so surprising. We have been thinking about God's memory of us. His remembering is active; it has a purpose, and it continues. When the people of Israel were enslaved in Egypt, God told Moses, "I have heard the groaning of the people of Israel ... and I have remembered my covenant ... I will deliver you" (Exodus 6:5-6). Remembering his covenant means that he will fulfil the promises that he has made.

In today's passage, Isaiah passes on God's promise once again to his people: "To grey hairs I will carry you". These people have been disobedient. God calls them "transgressors ... stubborn of heart" (Isaiah 46:8,12). Yet he loves them; they are his children, whom he has carried from before their birth. He will continue to carry them, right to the end.

In the Nativity story, when Jesus' mother Mary thinks of the baby to be born to her and "magnifies the Lord", she celebrates God's mighty actions and the "remembrance of his mercy" (Luke 1:46, 54). And Zechariah, celebrating the birth of John the Baptist, thanks God for fulfilling his promise to "remember his holy covenant" (v 72).

God remembers each one of us at every stage of our lives: not just in our "prime"—not just during the times when we feel we are able to serve with the most energy. He has "made" us, and he will always "bear" us (Isaiah 46:4), making up whatever we may lack. His Spirit is always in communion with our spirits, transcending cognitive limitations. And he makes plans for us in love: "I will carry and will save."

Daniel's wife, Phoebe, was living with Alzheimer's, which meant that for the last three years, her world shrunk down to their bedroom and en-suite bathroom, where she felt safe and secure. Daniel felt that they experienced many examples of God's grace and mercy in those years, particularly in Phoebe's main carer, Olivia, who came through a secular organisation. "She is a wonderful Christian, who, through her commitment, gave Phoebe an extra three years of life. Olivia even slept on the floor beside Phoebe's bed for the two nights before she died."

For some, the thought of going into a care home is hard. But many have found that they continue to experience God's love and care there. We don't know how the future will turn out. But we can be sure that God will remember his promise and will carry us and those we love to old age and beyond.

Reflect

What are your worries for future care? Have you explored the different options? Do you have examples of God's care that you can bring to mind, either for yourself or for others you know?

Day 12

Love Wins

There is no fear in love ... perfect love casts out fear.

1 John 4:18

How do we keep on loving well?

Shoko and I knew our Father God was in control. Despite that, I was often worried, tense and afraid. "I am full of fear and anxiety," I wrote in my journal. Shoko was often confused, and her behaviour was erratic. Like many others in similar situations, I worried about whether she would be willing to go out each day; would she eat well, would she resist taking her pills, or would I be able to settle her that night? That bedtime process was so often difficult, and from afternoon onwards, it occupied my thoughts. I knew it wasn't right, but I felt quite lonely in my fears.

Sometimes Shoko was afraid too. "Shhh, there are some people downstairs. How will we get food for them?" she would say. Or she would worry about "that man" who was telling her to do things, sometimes threatening her or telling her she had done wrong. Once, as we came into the house, she was convinced that he was upstairs or that he would come in at any moment. I had a hard time to persuade her that he wasn't coming.

It's easy to be afraid when we can't predict how a person is going to react. But how much more might they be afraid when their world is confused and they genuinely don't know how people will treat them, or what will happen next, from day to day. An experienced carer commented, "If I'm scared of the person I'm caring for, then he's all alone."[23]

As caregivers, we know we're the ones who should be giving reassurance to that person, by the way we relate to them, by our constant care and love. They need *comfort* and warmth. They need to feel *attached*, *included* and *occupied*. They need us (and others) to keep on *affirming their identity*.

How could I overcome my fear and help Shoko with her fears? I remembered John's words in the Bible: "Perfect love casts out fear". But what did that mean for us in our situation?

When John said this, there were two great truths that he wanted to emphasise. First, we know what love is because God has shown us his love: "In this is love, not that we have loved God but that he loved us and sent his Son" (1 John 4:10). This perfect example of sacrificial love has been shown to us in the humility of our Saviour, Jesus. So then, "if God so loved us, we also ought to love one another" (v 11). We are able to love because "he first loved us" (v 19). Going back to the source of love for comfort ourselves is the best way that we can love others in turn.

I realised that I had to focus on Shoko and her needs. It wasn't about myself and my feelings. For her part, between her fears, Shoko was constantly full of affection and told me again and again how much she loved me. That was more than I deserved but very reassuring.

"Beloved ... if we love one another ... [God's] love is perfected in us" (v 11-12). When we receive God's love and love from others, it takes away our fear and self-centredness. We can love those we are caring for, and they are not alone.

Reflect

What does love demand from you today? How will you show it? And how have you found that "perfect love" enables you to overcome fear or selfishness or other difficulties?

Douglas's Story

A few years ago, my dear wife of 45 years was diagnosed with vascular dementia—the top left quadrant of her brain was dead. To start with, she accepted the diagnosis, but as time went by, she became so embarrassed by it, so belittled by it, that she did her best to totally discount it. When the doctor explained vascular-induced dementia to her, he told her that the veins in her head bringing blood to her brain were blocked, like a garden hose blocked from bringing water to the lawn, and consequently, the brain had died, like unwatered grass. Since then, she has been standing with her head under the shower every day and swears she no longer has dementia, despite the evidence to the contrary, because she has been "watering the lawn". And, because it is the top left "logical" quadrant of her brain that is damaged, there is no way that we can discuss the diagnosis of her dementia, let alone deal with it rationally together.

As a result, my wife refuses to get any further medical help, which might mitigate her dementia. She's not only forgetting things but how to do things. She is Greek but forgets what garlic is. She loves cooking for large gatherings but forgets how to cook her favourite dishes. She hides the shopping I bring home all around the house and then spends the rest of the day looking for it. The other day, she withdrew all the money she had in her bank account and lost the lot. But the worst thing for me is that we can no longer discuss our problems and decide on how to solve them together, as we have always done. I can remember one occasion, by some miracle, we did manage to do it, but it backfired big time. She forgot what we had discussed, and when I proceeded on the basis that we had come to a decision together, my dear wife, with whom I have had a relationship of deep reciprocal trust for all those years, accused me of trying to trick her. Even now, I weep to think she would feel that I would try to make a fool of her.

A friend whose wife died recently with dementia advised me to make sure I did something every day to bring my wife joy, whether she remembered it or not. I asked another friend, who has become a wonderful spiritual advisor, for advice. He said, "You only have to ask and answer one question every day: what does love demand? And do it."

Part III

When We Suffer, God Is With Us

Day 13

How Long?

How long, O LORD? Will you forget me for ever?

Psalm 13:1

"What is the prognosis for a person living with Alzheimer's? What is the usual number of years after diagnosis?" I asked our community dementia nurse.

"Two to twenty years," he replied. He saw my face and added, "That's not helpful, I know. Seven to eight years is probably a closer time frame. But everybody is different."

I asked a care-home advisor a similar question about what we could expect. "Everybody has their own journey" was the reply.

She was right; I have seen the range of differences myself—one friend declined very suddenly, within eight months; others continue to do so very gradually. Robertson McQuilkin, a college president, cared for his wife devotedly for 25 years.[24] And the same is true for many other chronic illnesses.

How long?

Sometimes we ask the question fearfully: will we lose someone we love too soon? At other times we may feel frustration: how much longer will this continue, with suffering both for the person we love and for us too? We ask the question and then feel guilty. We should be caring joyfully and unselfishly. We don't want to think of the end, but we can't help thinking about it.

"That's what is so difficult just now," Emily said to me. "We thought David was going to die when he went into hospital three months ago, and he came through. But now he is so weak. How long can it go on? Our children are finding it very difficult. And I am feeling so tired."

"How long, O LORD? Will you forget me for ever?" The writers of the psalms asked this question often. It's repeated four times in Psalm 13 alone. This is one of the many psalms of lament, in which the psalmists pray for deliverance of some kind—from enemies, national conflicts, sickness or personal discouragement. Here, David, the writer, is afraid that his enemy will ultimately defeat him. And it makes him feel that God is distant and has forgotten him.

It is surprising—almost shocking—that Jesus asked the same question:

How long am I to be with you? How long am I to bear with you? (Mark 9:19)

He had much greater reason to express his frustration. He had come right down to our level; he had to endure his disciples' failures and lack of understanding. And there was always the shadow of the cross in front of him. He spoke plainly about it several times (8:31-32; 9:30-32; 10:32-34), and it must have been constantly on his mind. If even the Son of God could ask, "How long?" perhaps we can too.

What was it that kept Jesus going? Part of it was his open communication with his Father. He acknowledged his situation to the Father, as well as to his disciples. Jesus' words and the psalms of lament are not expressions of despair but of faith. They are directed to God, in confidence that they will be heard and that prayer will be effective. As long as you are calling out to God, you are acknowledging that he is the one who can deal with your situation. It's also helpful to be able to share it with others.

Psalm 13 ends with confidence:

But I trust in your unfailing love;
My heart rejoices in your salvation. (v 5, NIV)

We don't know what had happened to the "enemy" in question. Perhaps he was still there, but David now had confidence that God had heard his prayer.

How long? We don't know, but we trust that he does and has not forgotten.

Reflect

Do you feel that you can express your frustrations to God, without shame? Is there anybody else with whom you could share your feelings?

Pray through Psalm 13, with your own questions and words of trust. Or you could say, "Lord, you know my frustrations … [mention them to God] … I'm grateful for the example of David and even more of Jesus who spoke openly about their pain. Thank you, because I can trust your unfailing love."

Jessica's Story

My parents made the decision to have my grandmother living with them. When she moved in, I don't think any one of us expected her to live for another ten years. So for 20 years, my mother was her primary carer, and for 20 years, dementia was pretty central to our family life. I was working close by for 14 of those years so helped out often and whenever I could. The anxiety, the muddle and the confusion, coupled with her being very mobile, made for a really hard early period.

So why did my mother do this? Why was she prepared, with my father, to have hoists put in and carers coming to help for a couple of hours morning and evening? Why was she prepared to have her life slowed down and often interrupted? Why did we get our hands dirty with toilets and baths and messy food? Often we did cry out, "How long, O Lord?" What was our motivation?

These Bible verses were key to us over that period:

Honour your father and your mother. (Exodus 20:12)

When Jesus saw his mother and the disciple whom he loved standing nearby, he said to his mother, "Woman, behold, your son!" Then he said to the disciple, "Behold, your mother!" And from that hour the disciple took her to his own home. (John 19:26-27)

Honour widows who are truly widows. But if a widow has children or grandchildren, let them first learn to show godliness to their own household and to make some return to their parents, for this is pleasing in the sight of God. (1 Timothy 5:3-4)

And let us not grow weary of doing good, for in due season we will reap, if we do not give up. So then, as we have opportunity, let us do good to everyone, and especially to those who are of the household of faith.
(Galatians 6:9-10)

Day 14

Where Are You, God?

*My God, my God, why have you forsaken me?
Why are you so far from saving me,
from the words of my groaning?*

Psalm 22:1 (compare Matthew 27:46; Mark 15:34)

These are some of the bleakest words in the Bible. David prayed them while facing an awful situation. Jesus also prayed this same prayer on the cross. The words of this psalm find an extraordinary fulfilment in Jesus' suffering, which went far beyond that of David.

We too may echo them as we face our own suffering.

Miriam gave up work to care for her mother, who had dementia. It was hard as her mother became very restless and kept wanting to go out, whether she was dressed or not. "I felt so lonely. After my husband, Santosh, had gone to work, I cried every day. In those days there were very few resources. I had nobody to tell me what I should do.

Sometimes I said things that I shouldn't have said—and afterwards I felt guilty. I wondered why this had happened to my mother. She was such a godly woman. Why did God let this happen to her?"

What else did Jesus pray while he was on the cross? We know that he spoke the words from this psalm and soon afterwards words from Psalm 31:5: "Into your hands I commit my spirit" (Luke 23:46). As he suffered, was he praying through the psalms, which he knew so well? We can't know. But the fact that Jesus prayed using lines from the psalms of lament encourages us again that God has given us these words of Scripture to express our own grief.

Thirteen of the psalms described as "A Psalm of David" have titles describing the background experience of David's life.[25] Almost all of them are linked to times of suffering and failure referred to in the books of Samuel. They give us a picture of David's journey through suffering to his eventual kingdom (where he was still sinful and needed to repent). We read about his "tears and wandering steps" as well as his "humility, trust in the Lord, and penitence".[26] Jesus spoke to his disciples repeatedly about his own suffering. He told them that he must suffer. Did he understand his role as the suffering and persecuted Messiah partly from his knowledge of David's suffering and eventual glory?

Psalm 22 takes us through horrific experiences, which, in a mysterious way, are fulfilled in Jesus' suffering. But its writer also expresses trust: "In you our fathers trusted ... and [they] were not disappointed" (v 4-5, GNT). Words of trust and pain alternate from verses 1 to 21. Then, while still apparently suffering, he can say, "I will praise you" (v 22). And he concludes with the confidence that "all the ends of the earth shall ... turn to the LORD" (v 27).

We can't fully understand why Jesus had to suffer as he did, but we know it was because of his love for us, taking all of humanity's guilt on his shoulders. We don't understand our own sufferings, but Psalm 22 helps to lead us, even in the midst of the despair, to trust.

Reflect

Do the words of David, and even more of Jesus, give you any reassurance? Do they help you to express your pain to God? If you can, make some simple statements of trust as you think of God's character, what he has done in the past, and what he has achieved for you through Jesus.

"This is my situation now. But I trust you because…"

Mary's Story
Mary shares some hard lessons from her experience of support while caring for her husband.

- Don't assume that someone who has had a medical career is better able to deal with Alzheimer's. Many have experience of treating patients with this disease but have not been trained to understand the practical implications.

- Don't assume that you will get practical help when you are referred to a specialist service and receive the diagnosis. We were referred fairly quickly to the Memory Clinic and received the diagnosis. Graham agreed to help with two research projects. But it was all at a medical level; it was assumed that we were getting support from a different service. In the end we were put in touch with a person who gave us practical information and regular support—until the funding for her post was withdrawn.

- Don't assume that your fellow church members have sufficient awareness of dementia to enable them to know how best to help both you and the one who is living with dementia. We were hurt when a person who had come to Graham regularly for encouragement and advice told him that he didn't feel he should continue, as Graham was no longer capable. He had looked up to Graham so much and now did not know how to handle this new situation, so he stopped talking. That was very hard. But, unfortunately, it was not unusual at the time, as many felt unable to understand and respond appropriately to those living with dementia.

- Don't assume that those closest to you will be able to deal with the shock of this diagnosis. We told our family in quite a matter-of-fact way and didn't realise the level of their bereavement and shock. Perhaps we could have handled it better. Our youngest daughter told us later that she just sat down and howled. "I can't believe it. My father... Where is God?" You need to travel together and learn together. The family compass has to be reset. Our family came to be a great source of help and encouragement.

- Don't assume that you are prepared. Even with the help of books, websites or advice, there will always be something which catches the carer by surprise. Every situation is different, and the disease is unpredictable. I still remember the shock when Graham first said to me, "Is your husband still alive? Shouldn't you be getting home now?" And there were other times when he would count the "people" sitting in the room with us. I would reason with him: "I can't see them", until I realised I had to enter his world. Nothing really prepares you for those things.

Day 15

Wake Up, God

Awake! Why are you sleeping, O Lord?

Darkness is my only companion.

Psalm 44:23; 88:18 (GNT)

Psalm 44 ends dramatically: *Wake up, God! Why are you asleep?*

God's people are in deep trouble. At the start of the psalm, the writer looks back to a glorious past when God was clearly with his people, protecting them (v 1-8). He "delighted in them" (v 3). But now it seems that God has rejected them. They are facing defeat and disgrace (v 9-16). As he wonders why this has happened, he is provoked to his bold challenge. Why doesn't God intervene? Is he sleeping? The whole community are in great distress.

In Psalm 88, we find an individual in equally severe distress. We don't know what has happened, but he is "full of troubles". He feels forsaken by God and cut off from his friends. "I am shut in so that I cannot escape" (v 3, 7, 8).

Reading their words, it could sound as though the psalms of lament are just complaining. "You have cast us off" (44:9, NKJV) even though "we have not forgotten you" (v 17). Do we deserve what is happening to us?

Why do you cast my soul away? Why do you hide your face from me? (88:14)

But these are not just complaints; they are prayers. The writers are speaking directly to God, not complaining about him. As we read their words, we can hear and feel their pain, and we are invited to walk with them. We realise that we are not alone in our own pain. We are given space to express our own negative feelings and experiences directly to God, pouring out our hearts to him.

Lament is "the voice of pain, whether for oneself, for one's people, or simply for the mountain of suffering of creation and humanity itself. Lament is the voice of faith struggling to live with unanswered questions, and unexplained suffering. God not only understands and accepts such lament; God has even given us words in the Bible to express it."[27] But as we express our pain, we also ask how God will intervene to help us. In many lament psalms, we hear the note of trust, confidence and sometimes praise as the situation is resolved. But what if that has not happened?

Psalm 44 ends with the psalmist still loudly calling on God to intervene. The situation is still dire. It is only the reference to God's steadfast love, at the very end, which gives any basis for calling out and expecting an answer. This unfailing love is based on God's covenant with his people.

But Psalm 88 does not even have that. It contains "no expression of hope or faith anywhere".[28] The last words are "Darkness is my only companion" (v 18, GNT).

Where is the psalmist's faith?

It's right here, in his continuing to speak to God while he is in darkness. He is speaking to "a God who can be touched by a broken soul, a soul that is real and not covering up".[29] He can tell this God about the pain in which he is living. *I cry to you, Lord,* he says (v 13).

When you read psalms like these, you realise that you can be crying and know that "someone is listening. Someone can feel what you feel. Someone understands. You do not have to express your praise or words of trust when you feel like shouting or blaming".[30] We know that God is listening even more than the psalmists knew, because Jesus told his disciples that God "will surely give justice to his chosen people who cry out to him day and night" (Luke 18:7, NLT). And he will go on listening.

Reflect

Do you face situations in which you feel helpless and hopeless, not knowing which way to turn? Do you feel that you can pour out your heart to God? Even your tears can be prayerful as you bring your weeping and wondering to him. So keep speaking to him.

James's Story

We don't do much emotion in my family, much less crying. So I think my mum only realised she was grieving the loss of my father when her sister died. My dad hadn't died, but he had passed slowly but very definitely into another world—an Alzheimer's world. Even at the time when he retired, my sister and I noticed a change in his cognition and mobility, but because he had been so mentally active, the doctors wouldn't name it for years, preferring to call it "cognitive degeneration" instead of anything more definite.

Looking back, something more definite would have helped Mum. It would have helped her face what was happening to her husband—her best friend (perhaps her only friend)—and prepared her. She was constantly in denial: if only he would remember, if only he would go back to the way he was before, if only we could do something, anything. But of course we couldn't. Reminders on bits of paper went unheeded. Verbal reminders became nagging. She was grasping for other diagnoses and treatment that made no difference. Frustration rose for both of them, and he couldn't remember why. She became like a turbo-charged Martha, rushing around trying to fix everything, when perhaps she might have been a little more Mary and just sat with him while she could.

It seemed inevitable that she would become his carer, but she bristled against it; she didn't want to be a carer—she wanted to be his wife. But neither could she accept carers into the home, perhaps because that would make so final the decline that was evident to all of us. Really, she had lost him several years before, but only when she finally couldn't cope and he went into a home was she prepared to reflect on her feelings. Only when her sister died could she name it: grief. And she wept. Like Jesus weeping for Lazarus, so she wept for her friend who had passed, even though he had not yet died.

For me, it seemed like a train crash unfolding slowly but inevitably. It seemed so unfair—was so unfair—that my mum and dad, who had served others all their lives, were now being robbed of this time together at the close of their lives. But I couldn't do anything about that.

Sometimes we just weep. It seems so sad and pointless, and it hurts. And Jesus weeps too. But Jesus didn't stay in that of place of grief. Only a few verses later, Jesus had raised Lazarus from the dead.

Day 16

Why Me? Why Not Me?

Why did I not die at birth? ... Why is light given to a man whose way is hidden, whom God has hedged in?

Job 3:11, 23

"All of it sucks," wrote a daughter caring for her mother with dementia.

Job said pretty much the same thing about his situation. In fact, he expressed himself much more strongly—he wished he had never lived. At the beginning of his troubles, he had stood very firm. But as his suffering increased, he asked the question that all of us ask: "Why?" And even more pointedly, "Why me?"

It's a natural question every caregiver asks at some point. We don't even have to be suffering ourselves; there is more than enough suffering around us. We think about all that we have learned about God—our loving Father—and we ask, "If God is supposed to be like that, how can the world be like this?"[31]

I look at my friend David, a brilliant scientist, husband, a father and a church leader, who has wasted away physically and mentally, and I think, "Why?" Not everyone living with dementia is in that kind of condition. Many have great abilities and live with joy. But still we ask why.

Of course, there are other approaches to this question.

Arthur Ashe was the first African-American tennis player to win the men's singles titles at Wimbledon and the U.S. Open, and the first African-American man to be ranked as the No. 1 tennis player in the world. He contracted Aids through a blood transfusion and eventually died aged 49. When a fan asked him why God had chosen him for such a terrible disease, he replied, "When I was holding a cup, I never asked God, 'Why me?' And today in pain I should not be asking God, 'Why me?'"[32] "If I were to say, 'God, why me?' about the bad things, then I should have said, 'God, why me?' about the good things that happened in my life ... Now as I face my death, I can equally ask, 'Why not me?' Why not such a favoured person?"[33]

Arthur Ashe was right. In our fallen world, we experience both good and bad. Job bombarded God with questions and God didn't condemn him for it. But he showed Job that he couldn't expect to understand all the answers (as we see in Job chapters 38 – 42). We are not God.

But we still feel the pain. And as we lament, like Job, we are able to confront suffering. It is a reality for all human beings—a terrible reality for many. We cannot close our eyes or wish it away. Our lament can also become a means of growing in our intimacy with God, as Job discovered: "I had heard of you by the hearing of the ear, but now my eye sees you ... [I] repent in dust and ashes" (42:5-6).

It was not wrong for Job to ask questions; God commended him for his honesty. But Job assumed he had a right to know the answers. He had treated God as a distant third party whom he could call to account, but now God spoke to him directly. He was both reminded that God was greater than him and at the same time reassured that God still related to him personally.

Job's terrible experience led to new understanding and a deeper relationship with God. It is not dementia itself that helps us to grow; dementia is a terrible illness and it is difficult to say anything positive about it. It is our response to it and our experience of God that can bring about our growth.[34]

Reflect

What makes you ask, "Why?" What other questions do you have for God? Write them down. If you can discuss them with others, do so. Expressing yourself with honesty, like Job, is good.

What answers have you found? And what have you learned about God through your search?

Day 17

With the Three in the Fiery Furnace

*Did we not cast three men bound into the fire?
... But I see four men unbound, walking in
the midst of the fire, and they are not hurt.*

Daniel 3:24-25

For those of us who grew up in church, the story of Shadrach, Meshach and Abednego and the burning fiery furnace has inspired us since childhood. What conviction they had! They firmly believed that God would deliver them from this death sentence. Yet their words of faith included "But if not" (v 18). They decided that even if God chose not to deliver them, they would still refuse to obey the king's command. In many ways those three words are the most striking in the story.

But what amazed King Nebuchadnezzar was the appearance of a fourth person, seen walking with them in the furnace. This fourth man joined them in their fiery trial and brought them out.

When we suffer, who is with us? That's even more challenging than our previous question, "why?" Who is with us when we face the reality of dementia? Does anybody understand what we are going through? Do others know how it feels for the one living with dementia?[35] Do others realise how lonely we feel when the person we love is no longer with us, even though they are still here? They will never again be the person they were. We are alone.

Anthony cares for his wife, Irena, who has two rare forms of dementia. They affect her speech and vision, and because she can't find the words to express herself, she has withdrawn from meeting others or going to church. She loves gardening, but her work there is now chaotic. Her beautiful art has become darker and jagged. Anthony is committed to caring for her and works hard to find ways to occupy her positively. But he feels alone.

The story of Shadrach, Meshach and Abednego points us to an amazing truth. Just as the one "like a son of the gods" (v 25) was with the three in the fiery furnace, so Jesus, the Son of God, came to be with us humans in our fallen condition. He is with us today in whatever situation we find ourselves. And he understands because he has experienced all the sadness, temptations and pain that we experience. He is not "unable to sympathize with our weaknesses ... he learned obedience through what he suffered" (Hebrews 4:15; 5:8).

The Gospels describe Jesus' emotions, from overwhelming sorrow in Gethsemane (Matthew 26:38) to being filled with joy (Luke 10:21). He was witty and sometimes sarcastic, especially with his opponents. He used repetition and exaggeration to hold attention. A lot of it would have been humorous to his original hearers. But we also read that he shed tears (Luke 19:41); he was grieved, angry, frustrated, sorrowful (Mark 3:5; 8:21; 14:34). He was astonished (Luke 7:9; Mark 6:6) and distressed (Luke 12:50). The word actually means "constrained", "tense" or "stressed". It's amazing to think that Jesus too could be stressed.

Perhaps the commonest expression of his emotion was compassion—for a man with leprosy; for the crowds, like helpless sheep; for a widow who had lost her only son (Mark 1:40-41; Matthew 9:36; Luke 7:13). If he had met people living with dementia or their family and friends caring for them, he would have responded with compassion.

All these examples tell us that he genuinely experienced our human life. He understands what we are going through because he has been through it himself. Somebody once said to me, "I don't have to explain about our experience with dementia; you understand because you have been through it yourself." That might be true in a small way about you or me. But it is completely true about Jesus. When we suffer, he is with us in the furnace. He has been through all our experiences and more. We don't have to try to make him appreciate how hard it is; we can simply tell him how we are feeling. We know he will not judge us because he understands.

Reflect

What are some of the difficulties in your present situation—do you think that Jesus could have experienced the same kinds of things? Imagine his compassion towards you. How does that affect your praying?

Anthony's Story
My wife, Irena, was formally diagnosed with Alzheimer's PPA Logopenic variety (naming) in 2022. We celebrated our 30th wedding anniversary this week.

NOVEMBER 2022
Discontinued taking donepezil medication due to its rendering her into a zombie-like status all day long.

FEBRUARY 2023
Irena came out of the toilet at the airport and did not see me. Too late I realised she had gone astray. I discovered the airport was huge; it was over a kilometre to our gate—the final gate before a blank wall. I raced there, arriving one minute before it closed. To my astonishment and delight, Irena was there. I have never been so happy to see her lovely face. She said she did not know how she had got there. I am sure she simply walked until she got to the wall, and it just so happened that the gate was there! Thank God!

My wife and I are shackled together from now on. No travel except together. If I lost her in a crowd, I do not know how we would ever meet again. I now carry her travel pass, and her bank card is redundant because she can't remember her PIN.

FEBRUARY 2023
Irena woke looking and sounding dismayed and unclear about which way is up. She refused to go to church even though last week she was happy to go and received hugs, loving and caring behaviour, and complete acceptance.

Irena thinks she recognises strangers in a restaurant or train station; she says they were on the plane with us two weeks ago. She is also convinced that the neighbour is changing external plumbing to exploit us in some way.

MARCH 2023

"I don't even have enough vocabulary to speak to myself," Irena said.

Her world has become very small. She makes herself busy around the house but tends to wash clothes over and over again because she's a busy person with no idea what to do.

Irena's eyes look blank where once they were sharp and lively. I don't recognise my wife's face any more. The light is going out of it. This has been going on for at least a year now, but it's more pronounced.

Irena: "I feel I am coming to the end of a phase, and I don't know what the next one will be."

Me: "I love you, and I'll be with you, and we'll face it together."

AUGUST 2024

God bless my wife—my treasure on earth—who brought me to God, who shows integrity at all times, and who is always completely authentic. She often leads us in prayer and always starts by thanking God joyfully for what we have. May God bless her every day and give her a sense of real self-worth, and let her know that she is loved and admired and that her opinion is valued.

Day 18

Death's Bite Remains

Jesus wept.

John 11:35

Why did Jesus weep? He knew that he would overcome death and see Lazarus alive again—and very soon. We are clearly told that he knew what was going to happen and he trusted in God's sovereign plan (John 11:4, 11-15). He even waited before going to Martha and Mary so that he could raise Lazarus for God's glory (v 6). He wanted his disciples to believe. So why did he weep?

Jesus knew God's purpose in Lazarus's illness and death. But when he met Martha and, especially, Mary, he was "deeply moved in his spirit and greatly troubled" (v 33). It says literally that he "groaned in spirit and troubled himself". He was filled with grief, anger and indignation; was he wishing that he had come sooner? Or disturbed by seeing the others' emotions? We don't know, but clearly

Jesus felt powerful emotions. It was not only sadness and pain but anger at death. Death is an enemy to God's original purpose for humanity. Paul described death as "the last enemy" that Jesus will destroy (1 Corinthians 15:26). He would make that possible only by his own suffering and death. Perhaps that thought was in Jesus' mind as well.

So Jesus wept. Though he would overcome death completely, he felt real pain in the face of it.

Theologian Michael Horton preached a sermon with this title: "Death's Sting Is Removed, but Its Bite Remains".[36] It's a striking phrase that expresses a powerful truth. Death seems so final. We realise that sense of finality when someone we love dies, even when we were expecting it—almost waiting for it. Speaking of those living with dementia, Nicci Gerard says:

Even though we say that people with dementia are "gone", are "not the person they used to be" ... what we discover when they die is that they were after all still alive. They were after all themselves.[37]

When our loved ones die, we may believe they are with Jesus, but what we actually feel is *She has gone. I'm alone.* Death is painful, and we never really lose the scars it leaves us with.

During the First World War, Edward Shillito visited those who had been terribly wounded and disfigured. He wrote a poem, thinking of Jesus showing his scars to his disciples after his resurrection:

Lord Jesus, by thy scars we claim thy grace.
Show us thy scars ...
The other gods were strong, but thou wast weak;

They rode, but thou didst stumble to a throne;
But to our wounds only God's wounds can speak,
And not a god has wounds, but thou alone.[38]

Only Jesus is the God with wounds. He overcame death, but he carries its scars for ever. We know that death has been defeated but, like Jesus, we still feel its pain.

James grieved with his mother as they watched his father slowly fading away into death: "We mourn my father's situation and his slow passing from this world now. But we know, and my mum knows, and I think somehow, somewhere he knows too, that this isn't the end of the story. We grieve now, but one day we will rejoice. Now he is fading from this life, but one day he will be renewed and reborn, not because of a dementia drug but because of the resurrection power of God."

Reflect

How do you feel when you think of Jesus' reaction to encountering death and sorrow? Can you imagine him feeling a similar way about your situation? What questions would you like to ask him about death?

Part IV

We Have a Hope Beyond This Life

Day 19

Going Home

*I am going ... to prepare a place for you ...
I will come back and take you to be with me.*

John 14:2-3 (NIV)

"I have to go home," Shoko said. "How far is it to Tokyo? How do we go—by train or bus?" The next evening was the same: "I have to get to Maebashi from Tokyo. But I'm not sure how to get the train. I feel quite lonely. I can see them calling me, 'Come here and relax with us'. But I don't know how to get there."

Increasingly she was thinking about her family in Japan and wanting to go and see them, though she was confused about how she would do it. She began to talk about it almost every evening, as we sat at the table, and sometimes began packing food and other things to take. It was unsettling for both of us. Her restless longing seemed impossible to satisfy, especially as travelling had now become out of the question.

"Going home" is a frequent longing for those living with dementia. Each morning, Annette speaks to her mother in New Zealand, where it is late evening, and at this time of day her father is always wanting to "go home". Perhaps it's part of the common "sundowning" experience, when a person becomes restless, and sometimes agitated or distressed, often in the later afternoon or towards the end of the day. Maybe they are tired or uncomfortable or even in pain. Wanting to go home would be a very natural reaction.[39]

What is "home"? A place where we feel secure and relaxed? Where we are loved and where we are with those we love? It could be an actual place that we remember or just an idea that we are longing for. Do we have a home like that—a hope that we can hold on to, in the face of dementia?

Before his death, Jesus talked to his disciples about going home (John 14:1-3). He was preparing to leave them, and they were troubled. To reassure them, he promised that there was plenty of room where he was going and that he was about to prepare a place for them:

I am going there to prepare a place for you … I will come back and take you to be with me. (v 2-3, NIV)

The disciples didn't recognise the way in which he was going to prepare their place. Through his death and resurrection, he would overcome sin, evil and death itself. He would offer forgiveness and open the way for a restored relationship with God. Then—and still in the future today—he would come back and take them to be with him (v 3). He would be the way for them to come to the Father (v 6). So they would always be at home with him.

Jesus' words are a wonderful promise to all his followers that our relationship with him continues, now and even beyond death. "You will see me," he said to the disciples. "Because I live, you will live also" (v 19). Jesus does not explain here directly how this will be. For now, we hold on to Jesus' promise that he has prepared a place for us and he will take us there. So we will always be with him. We are going home.

This is our hope, already. As we wait for its completion, how should we pray for those living with dementia and for ourselves? We certainly pray for the sense that he is with us, holding us now. We pray for as full a life as is possible, supported by God's people and all the resources that are available. We pray for hope in the midst of our difficulties. And we look forward to our eternal home with him.

Reflect

Do you, or the ones you love and care for, have the desire to be "home"? What kind of place do you think Jesus has prepared for us? In what ways can you sense God's presence with you now as well as in the future?

Should we Pray for Healing for Those Living with Dementia?

We start from the basic principle that it is good to pray for any kind of physical (or other) need. The Bible is full of examples of prayer for such needs, from Isaac praying for Rebekah to conceive (Genesis 25:21) and onwards. The letter of James gives explicit instructions for praying for the sick (James 5:13-18). Our prayer is based on the belief that all healing comes from God, who made us. God uses the natural healing power of our bodies and minds, as well as the help of medicines and doctors. There are also times when he intervenes directly, without them. Examples of all three abound, both in the Bible and in the experience of Christians around the world and in every age. These principles apply to any kind of illness.

In a culture where medical skill and technology are so advanced, we can easily forget that all healing comes from God, though the means may differ. Other cultures may be more dependent on prayer and may see God's direct intervention more often. But whatever the means, healing comes from God, so we pray. Our prayer should also recognise that God is sovereign and does not always work as we may expect or wish. We need to pray with faith but not presumption.

What about illness that is considered terminal? We are used to the tension when we pray for someone with cancer, for example, between asking God to heal them and recognising that their illness may be terminal. We may know of those who have recovered, unexpectedly, from serious cancers, while we also know those who did not recover. Here, all the more, we have to pray with faith but not presumption.

These days many kinds of cancer, and other diseases that were considered incurable, are regularly cured through medication and therapies. So our understanding of what is a terminal illness may change. We also understand, more and more, the power of our attitudes to affect any disease. Our minds and spirits have a profound influence on our bodies. (And it works the other way round as well.) So the whole question of healing and cure is complex.

How do we apply this to those living with dementia? We are told that there is no cure for dementia and the disease progresses, though that progress varies enormously. The disease primarily affects the brain, so the greatest impact is on cognitive functions, though other physical functions may also be affected. There are medications that can help to slow the progress of the disease but won't stop it. New medications can slow the progress even more, but only for those at a very early stage.

Because dementia affects the mind and attitudes, our attitudes to the person living with dementia are of primary importance. They can almost form part of their treatment. It is well known that the progress of the disease is linked to surrounding attitudes and relationships with others.[40]

For those living with dementia, there is a lot that we can pray for.

- For people to understand that we should all be loved and treated as persons, whatever our condition.

- For true hope, which will give real quality of life in the face of this illness.

- For the progress of the disease to be slowed and for all the treatment that will help to be accessible.

- For those caring to have all the love, patience and resourcefulness that they need.

- For those who do not yet believe, that they will understand God's love for them and so have hope.

Can we pray that they be healed? In other words, that the progress of their disease is completely stopped? It is very natural, and right, to pray for our loved ones to be healed, at the same time praying that we would have the wisdom to know how to deal with their needs, and the patience and strength to keep loving and caring.

George is a retired church minister. He was forced to retire eight years ago when symptoms of memory loss and confusion were diagnosed (with two scans) as mild cognitive impairment and then fronto-temporal dementia. At his diagnosis, he was left with the clear impression that this was the end. It was a "brutal" diagnosis, and he and his wife planned his life accordingly.

At that time, he was part of a group that prayed often for him. When he moved to another church, a group there also began praying for him, as part of their regular prayers for the sick. In the last few years, he has found that his symptoms have not progressed; in fact, they have improved, and he is not aware of them anymore. He has felt great hope in knowing that he was being prayed for.

Christine Bryden, who has lived for many years beyond the expectation when she was diagnosed, writes with hope, as well as great sensitivity, about her experience of healing through prayer.[41]

What do healings like this mean? We might wonder about diagnoses, especially with so many uncertainties in this area. But at the very least, it is a challenge to pray with faith for those living with dementia, at all stages.

Day 20

I Shall See Your Face

*As for me, I shall behold your face in righteousness;
when I awake, I shall be satisfied with your likeness.*

Psalm 17:15

"You cannot see my face," God told Moses very clearly (Exodus 33:20). But that didn't stop the psalm writers from constantly longing to see God's face:

*One thing have I asked of the L*ORD *...
that I may dwell in the house of the L*ORD
 *all the days of my life,
to gaze upon the beauty of the L*ORD *...
My heart says to you,
 "Your face, L*ORD*, do I seek." (Psalm 27:4,8)*

And they believed they would see it:

I shall behold your face in righteousness. (17:15)

Did they mean that metaphorically in this life, or in the life to come? The Old Testament writers' view of life beyond the grave was sometimes unclear, but there are several references to their real hope. It was based on the fact that they already had a relationship with the living God, which could not be ended by death. Psalm 16:10-11 expresses this confidence, and 49:15 declares that "God will redeem my soul from the power of the grave" (KJV). We have another pointer to this in the much-loved Psalm 23:

> *Surely goodness and mercy shall follow me*
>   *all the days of my life,*
> *and I shall dwell in the house of the* LORD *for ever. (v 6)*

I read these words with my friend Alan while he was in hospital and beginning to sink with Alzheimer's and other complications. As I finished reading, he looked at me and said, "Yes, that is our great hope".

By the time of Jesus, there was a clear belief in the resurrection of the dead, though not all held it. Jesus clinched the argument in his words to the sceptical Sadducees, who mocked the belief: "You are wrong ... you know neither the Scriptures nor the power of God" (Mark 12:24). Then Jesus quoted God's words to Moses, *I am the God of Abraham, Isaac and Jacob.* "He is not the God of the dead, but of the living" (v 27).

Around the same time as this, Jesus had stood by the grave of Lazarus and told his sister Martha, "I am the resurrection and the life. Whoever believes in me, though he die, yet shall he live" (John 11:25). He would overcome death decisively. Lazarus came back to life—but eventually he died again. Jesus would be raised from death and never die. And his followers too will pass through death to be with him for ever.

This is the faith that sustains us in the face of death. We have experienced God with us in this life. That relationship will continue, and one day it will be completed. Our real self, our inner person, continues because he holds us in his memory. And eventually he will raise our bodies too, so that our whole person will be in his presence. He is the God of the living, as Jesus said to the Sadducees.

Christine Bryden, living with dementia, wrote:

My creation in the divine image is as a soul capable of love, sacrifice and hope ... As I unfold before God, as this disease unwraps me, opens up the treasures of what lies within my multifold personality, I can feel safe as each layer is gently opened out ... I will trust in God, who will hold me safe in his memory, until that glorious day of Resurrection, when each facet of my personality can be expressed to the full.[42]

This is not just unending life—it is life with Jesus in a relationship that continues. So it is his face that we see, as we look for the God who cannot be seen. "He is the image of the invisible God," Paul says. And he is also "the firstborn from the dead" (Colossians 1:15, 18), who is with us as we move from this life to the next.

One day, we will see him face to face, and it will be glorious.

Reflect

How does this hope strengthen us now, in our present situation, and for the future? What questions do you have about life beyond this life? Write them down: we may discuss some of them in the next two reflections.

Day 21

The Weight of Glory

So we do not lose heart… For this light momentary affliction is preparing for us an eternal weight of glory beyond all comparison, as we look not to the things that are seen but to the things that are unseen. For the things that are seen are transient, but the things that are unseen are eternal.

2 Corinthians 4:16-18

What keeps us going when things are hard?

The apostle Paul's second letter to the church in Corinth reveals, more than any of his letters, the pain he experienced as part of his ministry—the unbearable "affliction" that had led him to despair (2 Corinthians 1:8) and his sense that death was at work in him (4:12).

I sensed a similar despair in Denis's experience of caring for his wife, who was living with dementia:

Please God, I am so done in… Help us Lord, please! These are very, very difficult days for us two again. The hope I had in the summer for future happy care for my Julie has since been cruelly snatched away … everything is back on just my shoulders—(once again). I have to go on; there is as yet no alternative, but I am afraid my remaining strength is now going too … there is no "magic" answer for us … Four years of total 24/7, without any meaningful break, has pretty much broken me.[43]

Like Denis, Paul felt his situation was impossible. Yet he said, "we do not lose heart". He saw it as only a "light momentary affliction" in comparison with the future that God had in store for him—"an eternal weight of glory".

When things are hard, it is this act of looking beyond the present to God's perfect future that enables us to continue. We look forward to the day when that future will be revealed. In another letter, Paul speaks of the "glorious liberty of the children of God" (KJV), when the whole creation will be set free from its present "groaning" and "futility" (Romans 8:20-22).

What we see in front of us now are our present difficulties and limitations. But, like Paul, we remember that God is working something good through them, which we may never see. He is working good for us and, perhaps through us, for others. God's purpose is for us to become more like Jesus, as Paul reminds us in verses 28-29—"to be conformed to the image of his Son". And he is working that out in the midst of our present "momentary affliction".

So we continue with hope. We pray, and we help each other to live life to the full, helping to treat those living with dementia with our love and care. And whatever happens now, we have the assurance that we can look forward to what God has in store in the future.

What gives us that hope? We will see Jesus one day and continue our relationship with him. The writer to the Hebrews reminds us that Jesus endured the suffering of the cross "for the joy that was set before him". He is our example: the pioneer who has gone ahead of us on the road of suffering and has now reached the goal, his position of glory with the Father (Hebrews 12:2). So we are to "run with endurance the race that is set before us, looking to Jesus, the founder and perfecter of our faith" (v 1).

Denis realised the importance of holding on to Jesus and looking forward to what lies ahead:

> *My comfort is that my Saviour knows …*
> *His hands of compassion still hold us both.*
> *With my right hand I reach out to Him for strength,*
>   *day and night.*
> *My left hand grips Julie's all the time,*
>   *as she dozes each day.*
> *We await the days to come.*
> *Some are known only to me, none to my Julie.*
> *He knows them all, and will lead us gently on*
>   *until the very end.*[44]

So we keep looking to Jesus and the eternal weight of glory.

Reflect
Do you find yourself looking only at "the things that are seen"? What would help you to look to "the things that are unseen"?

Ajith's Story
Ajith Fernando learned from the experience of his friend Suri about the temporary nature of this life and the importance of the eternal.[45]

On 13th January 2018 at the age of at the age of 71, Suriyakumaran Williams went to be with the Master he had served so faithfully and lovingly. He had battled Alzheimer's disease for eight years.

When Alzheimer's was beginning to affect Suri, he continued to come to our accountability-group meeting until he lost the capacity to be at such a meeting. Each of us would have a time of sharing about how we were faring. Suri always shared the same thing: what he did for his devotions. He had had a consistent time of Bible reading and prayer all through his journey with God. He followed the example of the psalmist who said, "But I, O LORD, cry to you; in the morning my prayer comes before you" (Psalm 88:13). And that devotional time was still the fuel that pumped through his engine. But the time came when he did not have the capacity even to have a devotional time. When we visited him, he could not converse with us in any coherent way. We would end the visit with a prayer, and then he would interject with "Amen" and "Yes, Lord". Prayer still had a place amid diminishing mental ability.

But the time came when even prayer did not make sense to him. He was lost to earthly awareness. How often I asked God why he let this happen to his faithful servant. Always, the answer I got was that from eternity's perspective these years of sickness would be gloriously insignificant. Here, too, Suri spoke to us through his life.

And in his last sickness, too, he was teaching us. His utter helplessness pointed us to his ultimate destiny of heaven, where his service would be rewarded and consummated. It is good sometimes to be reminded of the temporary nature of life here on earth.

Day 22

Not as She Will Be

Then I saw a new heaven and a new earth ... God himself will be with them ... He will wipe away every tear from their eyes, and death shall be no more, neither shall there be mourning, nor crying, nor pain any more, for the former things have passed away.

Revelation 21:1-4

"I feel sad that my mother is not as she used to be," said our daughter.

"Yes," our vicar replied. "She is not as she used to be, and not as she will be."

What will we be like, in our new life beyond the grave? What will heaven really be like? The Bible gives us surprisingly little detail. The fullest description is in the last two chapters of Revelation (21:1 – 22:5), where John sees "a new heaven and a new earth".

He is showing us our final, permanent home. The old earth, with all its problems and its suffering, will be gone. The new heaven and earth are described as a real place. Like Jesus' resurrection body, their features have continuity with the present—buildings, jewels, water, trees with leaves and fruit (21:10 – 22:2). But they are also quite distinct—no more tears nor death, no more "mourning, nor crying, nor pain" (21:4). Peter's second letter calls them "new heavens and a new earth in which righteousness dwells" (2 Peter 3:13).

We can call this place our home because at its centre is love. That is what turns a dwelling place, however big or small, into a home. John describes an intimate relationship of love between us and God. In Revelation 21:3 he repeats three times in quick succession that God will be dwelling together with us. And he uses imagery of the church as a bride in verses 2 and 9.

We will be together with God, in relationship with him. This has been a central theme of our reflections, just as it is a central theme of the Bible: God with his people, from the beginning—"I will take you to be my people, and I will be your God (Exodus 6:7)—to the end, here, in Revelation: "He will dwell with them, and they will be his people" (21:3). The relationship continues.

What about those whom we love? Will we see them again?

The focus here in Revelation is on our relationship with God. That is the centre. Without that relationship, there is no future, no hope. But it is always implied that "we" will relate to God—not just individuals but together as a body of believers. The apostle Paul addresses this directly when he comforts the Thessalonian believers about their believing loved ones who have died (1 Thessalonians 4:13-18). When Jesus returns, God will "bring with him those who have fallen asleep" (v 14). Those who are still alive will be "caught up together with them", and all of us will "always be with the Lord" (v 17).

We will be together with those believers in Jesus whom we love. But will we recognise each other? Which version of a person will we see, especially if we have seen them change drastically in the present, perhaps through their illness? One thing is sure: love will connect us. Wendy Mitchell tells her daughters that one day, when her illness has progressed, "I won't know your names, but I'm sure I'll feel that emotional connection of love that we have for each other". And she wants them to know that "even though I won't recognise them, I still love them."[46]

We don't know much of the detail about our life in heaven; we would struggle to understand it in our limited state now. But we know we can look forward to being with Jesus, in our joyful permanent home, together with those we love.

Reflect

How do you imagine life in the immediate presence of Jesus? What questions do you have about that life?

Which Person Will We See in the Resurrection Life?

When we remember people who have died, we recall them at different ages and stages in their life. We are quite likely to remember them near the end, when their personality might have changed a lot through age or the impact of dementia or another illness. Or perhaps we think of them at a much younger age. Or from the years in between. But which one will we meet in the resurrection life?

1 Corinthians 15 is Paul's major reflection on the resurrection in general and, in particular, the resurrection body (v 35-57). We will have a new body, he argues, just like a flower or grain growing from a seed. The new body comes from the old—it is connected to it—but it is radically different as it has come through death.

So we are not to think of people as being just the same as they were here on earth. The resurrection life is in a different dimension altogether. "We shall all be changed", by God's supernatural power and according to his will—both those who have already died and those who are alive when Christ returns (v 51-52).

Jesus' appearances after his resurrection give us pointers to this new body. On the one hand, it was very different: he could appear and disappear at will; he was sometimes hard to recognise. But it was a real body, still able to be touched and able to eat and drink. He could be recognised, and he could communicate. There was no doubt about who he was.

Christine Bryden's reflection on her future resurrection body refers to her "multifold personality" and her trust in God as she waits for "that glorious day of Resurrection, when each facet of my personality can be expressed to the full."[47]

When we look at pictures of people we have loved, we usually have a collection from different parts of their life—perhaps from when they were very young, or from whenever we first met them, to when they were older; we see them with others, in good health and in bad health. We visualise all these stages.

In the resurrection life, I believe we will see the whole person, fully expressed—from all the stages of their life and all the aspects of their personality—and seen as fully integrated: the person as they really are, now transformed in the new resurrection body. It's a beautiful idea. If you wonder how that could be, remember Paul's words—it is "a mystery" (v 51)—and also Jesus' words, "You do not know ... the power of God" (Mark 12:24, NIV). Our God makes "all things new", including time (Revelation 21:5).

In her book *What Dementia Teaches Us About Love*, Nicci Gerrard imagines people she has known, after their death. She sees them now set free from the limitations that dementia laid upon them. In particular, she sees her father, who can now "walk around his garden, watering the tomatoes in the green house, pruning the roses and feeding the small brown songbirds. He can tie knots deftly ... sail a boat ... tease his grandchildren ... laugh with friends ... hold my mother's hand."[48]

She sees his whole personality and all the stages of his life that she knew. For Nicci, these are memories that she has beautifully brought together. But for those who believe in resurrection life with Jesus, these will be realities. When

Amy Carmichael, a mission leader in south India, was nearing death, she wrote these words about her hope for her beloved adopted daughter, who was also dying:

Tell her that after I see His Face the first face that I shall want to see will be hers, and for ever and ever we shall be together.[49]

We have to be a bit cautious with what we imagine, as there is so much that we have not been told. But one thing we know for sure is that Jesus is the only one to have come back from the world of the dead to glorious eternal life. He conquered death and inaugurated the resurrection life. As we look at him, we have a glimpse of what that will be like.

God's purpose for us is to become more and more like Jesus. We trust him to fulfil this in us all, even when faith and understanding may have become uncertain because of dementia. One day his purpose will be complete. And as we come closer to him, we will come closer to each other.

Part V

We Are Part of a Loving Community

Day 23

You Did It to Me

Whenever you did one of these things to someone overlooked or ignored, that was me—you did it to me.

Matthew 25:40 (MSG)

Caring for others is part of our vocation as human beings. From the beginning, God gave the first human beings the task to care for the world and its creatures. It is a broad mandate for the whole of creation. But at the centre is care for each other, and particularly for those in any kind of need.

Jesus brought this mandate into very sharp focus in his parable of the last judgment (v 31-46). The "righteous" show their care by responding, perhaps unselfconsciously, to people in any kind of need. All of us have the challenge and privilege of caring for one another in different ways, whether we are family members, friends or professional carers. But Jesus shocks us with this comment: "That was me—you did it to me" (v 40, MSG).

Unfailing Love

In other words, our attitude to others shows our attitude to Jesus. That lifts the task of caregiving to a whole new level. We may feel it is quite beyond us. But it does give a new dignity and purpose to what we do, however small. We are doing it for Jesus.

We can see those living with dementia among those who are "overlooked or ignored". For some, there is still a stigma attached to dementia—though it is slowly disappearing as awareness continues to grow. Some, especially those with young-onset dementia, may feel they have a significant contribution to make to our understanding of the disease, but they are not always listened to. Others, in later stages of the disease, are often ignored because they are seen as being difficult to communicate with.

Caregiving requires a high degree of ability to do it well. We could make a long list of skills that caregivers develop through their work: communicating, learning, decision-making, researching, collaborating, being flexible. And all of these exercised on the job, under pressure, without a break, and often in the face of great personal sadness.

But the most basic qualification for being a caregiver is not in this skills list. It is simply love, as we have noted more than once. We have received God's unfailing love, and we reflect that love to the ones that we are caring for. "With love you can make every day the best it can be," writes a caregiver.[50]

Earlier, we thought about the flower with different facets of love that Dr Tom Kitwood advocated, reflecting the needs of the person living with dementia. Anthony has made another checklist from his experience as a caregiver:

> *Carers' responses must be consistently and completely reassuring, positive, cheerful, with unwavering love, trust,*

kindness, gentleness, and self-control. Logic and argument have lost their effectiveness, so distract and divert instead. There is no room for impatience and frustration.

How do you manage to do that? Look at another list from the apostle Paul:

The fruit of the Spirit is love, joy, peace, patience, kindness, goodness, faithfulness, gentleness, self-control.
(Galatians 5:22-23)

You can see similarities to the first list; the qualities that the Spirit produces give us a pattern for caregiving. But when we feel there is no chance of reaching that standard, we need to remember that it is not a list of demands that we have to achieve. It is fruit that the Spirit grows in "those who belong to Christ Jesus" (v 24).

Jesus is the perfect example of all these qualities. And he is living in us by his Spirit; his life in us empowers us to become like him. He is producing the fruit of love within us—his own character growing in us as we trust in him. As caregivers, we are fulfilling our human vocation, but, more than that, we are expressing the life of Jesus in us. We are doing it for him.

Reflect

When you think about caregiving, do you think that you are doing it "to Jesus"? You may not see it on a day-to-day basis, but remember that his Spirit is producing the fruit of Jesus' character in you. Are there ways in which you can encourage that process? Which aspect is the most difficult for you?

Day 24

Clay Pots

But we have this treasure in jars of clay.

2 Corinthians 4:7

Caregivers have a high and wonderful calling. It can also be demanding. I remember receiving a note from a friend when I was trying to care for my wife:

It amazes me how the Lord invites us to love more and more deeply in ways we would not have thought of when we were younger ... Well done. You and Shoko are in my prayers.

I appreciated his words, but I didn't really want to accept this invitation from God. It was too challenging. I was too tired. But as I thought about it more, it was also moving and encouraging. It was a calling, and there was a purpose to it.

We have already looked at how the apostle Paul reflected on his ministry as he wrote to the church in Corinth. He had experienced affliction and despair (2 Corinthians 4:8

and 1:4-8); he had been misunderstood and falsely accused. Despite that, he regarded his ministry of the new covenant as something splendid and glorious, shining "the light of the gospel of the glory of Christ" (4:4). He was literally holding treasure. "But," he said, "we have this treasure in jars of clay" (v 7). We are just clay pots: disposable, fragile, breakable.

When we lived in India, tea used to be served on train journeys in small clay cups. When you had drunk your tea, you just threw the cups away, beside the railway track, where they would disintegrate back into the ground. They were eco-friendly, cheap and completely disposable.

Paul's metaphor reminds us of what it means to have a calling. Unlike those clay cups, we are not disposable—we are valuable to God. But we are fragile. When we are crushed or knocked about, it hurts. We keep going because the focus is not on us but on our purpose—on the treasure we hold. Like Paul, we are shining the light of the gospel as we serve with patience and perseverance. We are doing it for Jesus' sake (v 11). And we are doing it like Jesus. He calls all his disciples to take up their cross and follow him: to "lose" our lives for his sake (Mark 8:34-35).

We may feel that we are failing in our calling. We are very aware of our limitations and sometimes our unwillingness. But God uses our imperfections to deepen his work in us. The Sri Lankan leader who taught me about lament and faith (Day 7) wrote something else about what he had learned:

My failures in ministry are partly responsible for whatever depth there may be in my ministry. Failure drives me to think, to theologise, to confess failure… to battle for patience and, most importantly, to depend on

God's grace. My failures have taught me so much more than the few successes I may have had along the way.[51]

The Japanese art of repairing broken pottery with powdered gold lacquer—*kintsugi*—has become well known. The cracks and imperfections become a source of beauty instead of disfigurement. As clay cups or jars, we may have plenty of cracks. God uses us despite our imperfection.

Reflect

Do you see your caregiving work as a calling? What difference would it make to your everyday experience if you saw it in that way?

Day 25

We Need Friends

They came [to Jesus], bringing to him a paralytic carried by four men ... And when Jesus saw their faith, he said to the paralytic, "Son, your sins are forgiven."

Mark 2:3, 5

When the paralysed man could not move, his four friends picked him up and carried him to Jesus. And it was their faith that Jesus recognised when he healed the man, both spiritually and physically.

The main point of this story is Jesus' words of forgiveness, which provoked hostility from his opponents and demonstrated his authority as "the Son of Man" to forgive sins. His words and actions had a powerful impact on everybody there (v 10-12).

That makes the friends' actions all the more remarkable; it was their faith that enabled their friend to receive Jesus' help and enabled Jesus to show his authority. When people need

Jesus' help but feel only their weakness and lack of faith, we can support them. Each of us can look out for others who may be struggling physically, emotionally or spiritually. Friends can exercise faith on behalf of others. They can pick them up and carry them through difficult times.

People living with dementia particularly need others to "hold their story" as Tom Kitwood puts it—people to maintain continuity with the past and keep them going.[52] As caregivers, we can help to preserve their sense of identity and all that is important to them, in the face of an illness that is trying to strip them of these things.

But caregivers can't do it alone. We are the ones under constant pressure, sometimes discouraged despite our efforts. And that is why friends are so important, both for the person living with dementia and for caregivers. A friend can give practical help across a range of areas and, even more importantly, they can give the gift of their time by keeping in touch.

But friends don't always find it easy. They may feel their old friend with dementia has changed so much, perhaps not recognising them anymore. They are not in regular contact, like caregivers, so they may become discouraged and wonder if it is worthwhile. Christine Bryden addresses friends and family of those with dementia, speaking from her own experience:

> *Try to realise that it is not important that we remember that you visited us, for it is the experience of Christ's love that you bring us, not a memory of an event ... does it really matter that a few hours later we will have forgotten that you have given of yourself and brought the Christ-light to us?*[53]

Jessica found that some of her relatives couldn't cope with the change that dementia had made to her grandmother:

One of my cousins said to me, "She isn't the same person anymore. I would rather remember her as she was, so I won't visit her now." That made me sad and angry. We must embrace and help those who are faced with this scary and difficult condition. Hugs, hand-holding, remembering the past, sitting close by—they all help that person to feel loved and still needed and wanted. It isn't about whether the person remembers us. It is about us showing something of God's unconditional love and kindness.

As caregivers, we can get so caught up in the intense caring role that we become isolated too. We also need the affirmation and support of friends. One important need is friends with whom we can talk in confidence. I used to meet our vicar for an hour every three weeks. He listened without judging as I expressed my difficulties, frustrations and, sometimes, doubts. He asked questions about my wellbeing, and we prayed together. It was a lifeline. If we don't already have somebody like this, it's something important to pray for.

The church is, above all, a community of love and friendship. Whether we are primary caregivers or less closely connected but concerned for our friends, can we be like the four who brought their friend to Jesus? It wasn't easy! They faced real obstacles, but their love and faith enabled them to be bold and creative. And it was their faith that brought healing of body and spirit to their friend.

Reflect

Do you have somebody you can talk to in confidence about the challenges you are facing? Or to help with the practical burdens? If not, could your church help you to find somebody? Ask God to bring the faithful support you need.

Sushila's Story

While my sister-in-law, Ritu, was still able to walk, her husband used to take her out for a walk each day. After some time, he needed to hold her hand and guide her. Eventually she needed two people to accompany and support her, with a wheelchair in reserve.

If she met a friend while out, her eyes would light up, and she would hold out her arms to embrace them. But some would ignore her when they met, talking only to the other person with her. Others whom she used to meet regularly stopped contacting her.

Her friends didn't understand what had happened to her and probably felt awkward about how to communicate. This kind of early-onset Alzheimer's was still quite rare. If I was with her, I tried to tell them that it was important to go on talking to her, even if she didn't answer. She was still their friend, I said, and she appreciated their contact.

Day 26

All Things in Common

All who believed were together and had all things in common ... There was not a needy person among them.

Acts 2:44; 4:34

Imagine being part of the early church with its intense community life. It wasn't only that they shared their possessions—though that was remarkable. They shared their whole lives as they prayed and praised God together. Their "glad and generous hearts" (2:46) encouraged each other and impacted their community. Nobody felt discouraged in that setting, so much so that "there was not a needy person among them" (4:44).

What would that look like today for families affected by dementia?

"My family didn't understand," said Rachel, who cared for her mother for ten years. "They only visited from time to time, so they didn't see her real situation."

"My sister and I supported our mother in very different ways," Claudia remembered. "Sometimes my sister told me I didn't really care."

Families can be divided as they try to respond to the chronic, terminal illness of someone they love. All of us have different ways of coping. This is a challenge for the church. We are called to be together—to have "all things in common". We are supposed to be a family. But, as in a human family, we don't always know how to get it right.

Living with dementia and caring for a person living with dementia are strange situations. The disease may come in stages, sometimes not noticeable at all—it doesn't fit into neat categories. Acknowledging it openly is difficult for some. At what point do we speak about it? There are no rules; as in any relationship, the people involved need respect and sensitivity. Those of us who are affected may be reluctant to ask for help or even to acknowledge our situation. And others may feel ill-equipped and unsure about how to relate to us. They are afraid of making mistakes.

But the early church's example suggests we can be more open and intentional. Some churches have set up groups to provide this encouragement; others may have more informal ways to find out about needs and offer support. A page on the church's website is helpful. When we know that others recognise our situation and really want to know how to help, it is genuinely encouraging.

Building these relationships works both ways. When I was finding my caring role challenging, a friend at church asked me, "How are you?" and I just replied, "I'm fine, thanks," without any thought. Later I realised he really wanted to know because he knew a bit about my situation. I went back and apologised for my superficial reply. It led to a good conversation and a much deeper relationship. As I acknowledged my need, I was able to receive his encouragement.

When you are the one in need, it is hard to have the energy to ask for help; it is much easier when others anticipate our problems. But we shouldn't hold back from being honest with others, as well as with God, about our personal needs. Sometimes people need more help to know what is the best thing that they can do for us.

Having "all things in common" might not mean sharing our money (though it might). But it does mean sharing our time and thought and practical concern so that there is "not a needy person" among us (Acts 4:34). Rather, any of us caring for friends or family members will know we really are supported and held "together".

Reflect

Does your church have ways of supporting you as a caregiver? What would you like to see it do more or better? Write down your suggestions and pray for ways to share them with your church.

The Barnabas Group

After her husband died, Jane wished there had been a supportive group that they could have joined within their church. So she began one herself.

With the help of a friend, we began meeting in my home with those already affected by dementia, to share information and to pray together. As we identified more and more people who needed this, we switched to a venue at church with encouragement from our clergy team. We then planned a one-day dementia awareness conference. It was well attended, not only from our church and town but also from further afield.

Our monthly support group continued to reach more people who were affected, and we named it the Barnabas Group, indicating our desire to be a source of encouragement to others in need. We share information, sing and pray together, enjoy refreshments and enjoy some activities. We try to engage the interest of our members and evoke memories that they can share. We welcome any who wish to join us. Some come with carers, but some live alone, and our team members pick them up. Some spouses use the Barnabas time as respite from their caring.

We felt the need for a more accessible worship service and, with our vicar's support, a short monthly midweek service began in the smaller chapel area of our church. We print a new booklet for each service with the words of the hymns, prayers (using some that are familiar from the past) and our Bible-reading. Our members can take it home. Every second month we include a shortened communion service. Wednesday Worship has been given such a welcome, and it also appeals to those who find a long service difficult or who are cut off for other reasons from Sunday services.

Alongside all of this, we try (with a growing team of helpers) to support those who are caring for their friends and family living with dementia. We believe we can constantly remind each other that we are not alone, we have the strength and help of our God, and we have hope for the future, no matter how hard the present may be.

For more information about the Barnabas Group and how it's run, visit **allsaintscrowborough.org.**

Day 27

When One Member Suffers...

If one member suffers, all suffer together; if one member is honoured, all rejoice together. Now you are the body of Christ and individually members of it.

1 Corinthians 12:26-27

How do we know which members of the body are suffering or being honoured, and how do we join with them? In Paul's metaphor of the body, all the parts are closely connected, and we can feel that easily. But when we think of those living with dementia, and their family and friends, it may not always be obvious. As caregivers, we know that we need to find all the resources that are available. And we would love to have others who could support us in our task. But we don't always find it easy to let others know about our situation and to communicate what we actually need.

Christine Bryden encourages caregivers and those with dementia alike to move "towards becoming a care-partnership, in which we accept, collaborate and adapt to new roles within the journey of dementia". She describes someone with dementia as "an active partner in a circle of care."[54] Another name for a circle of care is a support team—a group that gathers round a person living with dementia and their caregiver(s) to give them ongoing support and encouragement. You may already have a good support network, or you may be struggling, feeling that you are on your own.

I remember meeting a friend at a time when Shoko's situation had taken a sudden dip. I was exhausted—not sure which way to turn. Our friend took one look at us both and said, "You need support! You can't do this on your own." She was right, but it took time and effort to build the team. We needed the professionals (e.g. medical, social services, paid carers), but it was hard work to navigate the range of different resources when they didn't always seem to be joined up.

We also needed our family and friends, including our church. We couldn't have survived without them. They helped to fill what broadcaster and author Sally Magnusson calls the "empty centre" of dementia care.[55] But we had to work out how to let people know about our situation and then what kind of support would fit best. Someone offered to take Shoko out for a drive without me to give me time off, but that wouldn't have worked. Coming to our home to visit and spend an hour with her, in her familiar setting, did work well.

It takes openness and sensitivity on all sides to build an effective support team. If our church is going to be a place where we truly "suffer together" and "rejoice together" with other members of the body, we need to build open, trusting relationships. We may need to learn better how to communicate. As caregivers, we can discover the value of inviting others who have greater emotional distance from our situation to enter the reality of our dementia world. Sometimes they can help by bringing a different perspective.

Tim's wife, Jean, was doing her best to adjust to his changing ways with dementia, but trying to understand what was going on in his mind wore her down. A friend at church, Sue, was aware of her situation and introduced them to Richard, who began to visit Tim regularly. They would go for a walk and a coffee, giving Jean time on her own. Tim opened up to Richard about his hopes and concerns, and he was able to reassure him. It made Tim more relaxed, and it was a relief to Jean that somebody else could support them. Sue and Richard had become part of their support team.

We are supposed to suffer together. Paul reminds us in 1 Corinthians 12 that God has appointed us all with different skills, roles and parts to play within the body. These may change at different points in our lives, but all are vital. Paul says that there should be "no division in the body, but that the members may have the same care for one another" (v 25). We need to know each other's situation so that we can offer this. You may feel more comfortable with giving, but there is also a time for receiving help from your brothers and sisters in Christ. We are not a burden on each other—rather, as members of the same body, we give and receive, suffering and rejoicing together.

Reflect

Do you have a support team or "circle of care"? List some of the ways they are supporting you. If not, do you think your church members can help you to develop one? Can you communicate your situation to a church leader? What would you most like people to pray for you?

Clare's Story

Clare cares for her mother living with dementia, along with her sister who lives much closer to her. For Clare, it's a two-hour journey each way, two or three times a week, which is demanding.

I love to see my friends, but I've told them, "I haven't got the emotional space to think about meeting up. If you were to knock at my door, I'd be very happy. But please don't ask me to plan. You can't rely on me to sort it out right now."

I have a good friend who supported her parents, and she gets it. She just says, "Right, are you free on this day to come over?" And that's easier because she's done all the organising. I used to be very hospitable, but now there's a reversal of roles.

The best people are the ones who have been caring themselves (or are still caring). One friend comes over to me in church, and she doesn't just ask, "How's your mum?" She says, "How are you, Clare?" And I say, "Well, you know…" And she replies, "Yes, I know". She just understands me—and I haven't told her anything or given her any details. But I think there has been a meeting of hearts.

Some people seem to think that if you are facing a new season of difficulties, you should drop all your other roles. And there's a part of me that agrees—I've had to stop hosting the home group in my home—but I don't want everything taken away because I don't want to be completely consumed by care. I like to do other things and feel that I've got something to contribute.

I've realised that in my church, we are very good in a crisis, but not very good in supporting a long-term situation. We rally round in an emergency, but when something goes on and on and on you have to work a bit harder to see what's needed. I've had to accept that certain people will be there long-term, but others move on, even though your season continues.

Day 28

The Lord Will Keep You

I lift up my eyes to the hills.
From where does my help come?
*My help comes from the L*ORD*,*
who made heaven and earth.
He will not let your foot be moved;
he who keeps you will not slumber.
Behold, he who keeps Israel
will neither slumber nor sleep.
*The L*ORD *is your keeper;*
*the L*ORD *is your shade on your right hand.*
The sun shall not strike you by day,
nor the moon by night.
*The L*ORD *will keep you from all evil;*
he will keep your life.
*The L*ORD *will keep*
your going out and your coming in
from this time forth and for evermore.

Psalm 121

This was our family's "journey psalm", which we loved to read before long journeys or big transitions like starting at a new school, moving to another country or going for a job interview. It was the phrase "your going out and your coming in" that linked it to journeys for us. But this psalm is about the whole of our lives. We can always be sure of help from the Creator (v 1-2), who doesn't let us slip or fall (v 3), is always alert (v 3-4), protects us (v 5-7), guides our journeys and brings us safely home (v 8).

What is the most difficult journey? For some it might be the transition to a care home, or the thought of it. It can be an excruciating decision to make.

Fiona's mother needed to go into a home. It was clearly the right choice, for many reasons. But Fiona knew that her mother would have greatly preferred to stay with family, and so she carried a sense of guilt, even though there was no other alternative. It's an option that all of us may have to consider at some point as we care for one another. We each have to make our own decision according to the situation, trusting God for the outcome. It will never be an easy step, and for some the reality has been very hard too. But for many, it has proved to be an excellent solution. Families have found that our Creator God has provided just what was needed, because he is their "keeper". "He will keep your life," the psalmist says, reflecting the ancient blessing of the people of Israel—"The LORD bless you and keep you" (Numbers 6:24).

Some have to care at a distance. Amy's family live on the other side of the Atlantic, where her father was caring for her mother, who was living with dementia. When he suddenly died, the family felt they needed to find a care home for her. It has worked well, and she is settled there. But she has declined so much that she can no longer speak to Amy on FaceTime—it's too confusing. If Amy wants to see her and talk with her, she really needs to be with her physically. She would also like to be able to support her brothers, who live near their mother. But all these things require money and time for travel, as well as needing to factor in her responsibility for her own children. She prays for wisdom and strength, on the one hand to know how and when to visit, and on the other hand to release her mother into the Father's care. He will not let her "foot be moved", and he will "neither slumber nor sleep", so Amy can trust that he is caring for her mother even when she cannot be present.

As we face these huge life decisions, we ask, "From where does my help come?" Our Creator keeps us, whether day or night, whether out or in—wherever we are.

Reflect

Do you need to make decisions about care homes or other kinds of professional care? Use this psalm to bring your requests and concerns to God now. You can repeat it and ask your Father God to bring you peace through his promises.

Fiona's Story
Once my father died, my mother came to live with us. She was very arthritic; she used a walking frame and a wheelchair and was in considerable pain most of the time. My mother was a lovely, gracious lady with a deep faith and a kindly disposition, and had spent most of her life caring for others. She had painted beautiful pictures and sewn lovely embroidery until arthritis took over her hands. Her dementia had not changed her character, and she was still a delight to have around.

Producing meals and doing general chores for her was easy enough; help from my husband was great, visits from carers, the nurse and physiotherapist soon filled the day—but accompanying her for three or four toilet visits every night, each taking some 45 minutes, was a lot to cope with. While my mother dozed off during the day, I needed to be awake to do the domestic chores and to work from home, even occasionally going into the office. It was exhausting.

Everything came to an abrupt halt when, having had a small operation for breast cancer, it was decided that I needed chemotherapy and radiotherapy. So my mother went, willingly but temporarily, into a care home. As the months went by, I recovered, but my mother had become significantly less mobile, needing a hoist to move from the bed to a chair. Her doctor said that she was best staying where she was and that I should not be doing the caring after having been so ill. My mother would have greatly preferred to stay with family. Though she was beautifully cared for, she was no longer so happy. Not realising how much work it was to care for her, she could not fully understand why she couldn't come back.

My siblings were not in a position to help, though we all visited her. In the fourteen months that she was there before she died, hardly a day passed without one or more of us coming to the home.

But this situation was excruciatingly sad for us. My mother had lived a life of caring, and we were not able to return that care ourselves. Yes, the professionals were in favour of the decision. Yes, it made sense for different people to look after her different needs at different times of the day, and so be fresh and alert as they worked. Yes, even if I had not had a spell of illness myself, I would one day have had to admit that I could not cope, eventually setting aside my own pride. Yes, she probably was cared for in a safer environment by people who had the relevant skills. Yes, we prayed about all of this so much at this time. I still live with that sadness and sense of guilt.

It was a great feature of the care home that it was attached to the local church, and residents could be wheeled there in five minutes. We moved churches to become members there so that in church and in the hall afterwards for coffee (sometimes with friends she knew), she felt as if she was her own person rather than in an institution. We will be forever grateful for the love and care of the church members at that time.

Day 29

Love as I Have Loved

A new commandment I give to you, that you love one another: just as I have loved you, you are also to love one another.

By this we know love, that he laid down his life for us, and we ought to lay down our lives for the brothers.

John 13:34; 1 John 3:16

Jesus' love was sacrificial. He laid down his life, quite literally. Loving like Jesus means loving with our will. As John Swinton writes, "It requires determination, fidelity and an intentional desire to be with the other and continue to love."[56] That kind of love can be complicated at the best of times, and it becomes "even more complicated within the context of dementia, when personalities and behaviours can change and those whom we love can appear very different than they once did".[57] We are conscious of what we have lost in the relationship, and our feelings may be affected. But our intentional love continues even though its form may change.

We can look for joy in the things that we are still able to do together—perhaps walking around the supermarket, singing together, looking at photo albums (even after people can no longer be recognised), welcoming friends or joining with others in church each week. And when these simple things are no longer possible, we look for other ways to express our intentional love.

Jesus loved his disciples intentionally "to the end" (John 13:1), despite their weaknesses and frequent lack of understanding. Their love failed him many times. Soon after Jesus had washed their feet and taught them about living in love, in his time of greatest distress, the disciples fell asleep rather than watching and praying with him as he had asked (Matthew 26:36-46). Jesus loved with persistence and faithfulness; he is a constant example for us.

As caregivers, we may need to learn to love without necessarily being recognised or remembered in return. Christine Bryden described her way of responding to others, as a person living with dementia—not always as expected: "The way I know people is in a spiritual and emotional way ... right at their core. But I have no idea who they are, in terms of ... your world, of cognition and action, and labels and achievements."[58]

In displaying love, our body language is more important than our words. An impatient tone of voice or appearing to be in a hurry can cause distress—"Why are you so cross with me?" While an encouraging hand or a smile can bring a rewarding smile in return. When we love with intention, we are more likely to receive love back, even if the expression is weaker or sometimes barely recognisable.

I watched Kiran, a friend whom we had known for many years, when he came to visit. We had not seen him for a long time, and Shoko didn't remember him but realised he was somebody close to us. She welcomed him but was also disengaged. I was amazed at the intuitive way in which Kiran related to her, talking to her warmly and directly, not at all put off when she didn't respond. He connected with her, and I was deeply grateful.

Emotions and feelings do not die with dementia. "I'll always remember my grandmother at the end of a happy family day," said Jessica. "In her bedroom, she looked at me and said, 'I have had a happy day, haven't I? I can't remember what I have done, but I feel very happy.'"

"Caring for Ritu as a family has brought us all closer," said Sushila. "We have talked about end-of-life care and how we will face it together. On one occasion, Ritu woke up and said to her daughter, 'I love you'. The whole family was amazed, and we shared the impact together. Now even a single word is beyond her. But we know that the love remains."

Ray looked after his wife for many years as her mental capacity got worse. We admired him for his faithful and patient care. When she eventually moved to a care home, he continued to visit every day. "Why do you do it, when she doesn't recognise you?" a friend asked. "She doesn't know me," he replied, "but I still know her".

The forms of love may change, but the intention remains.

Reflect

What have you learned about ways to express your intentional love? How does Jesus' example motivate you? And what expressions of love have you also received?

Jessica's Story

My grandmother loved bedtime and being clean and cosy in bed. We always prayed with her and then sang. "Wide, Wide as the Ocean" was a hit, and she would always add the last word, "everywhere", at the end if you paused for her!

The last few years involved washing and feeding my grandmother, keeping her hydrated and maintaining the things that she loved most: having children around, hearing familiar hymns and songs, going to church every week and being in the midst of her family.

She had stirred the Christmas pudding a few weeks before she died, aged 99. She never stopped being in the thick of her family. She was valued to the end, and she taught us lessons which I do not want to forget—it's why I love helping out with the senior ladies at my church. I think we were very blessed as a family to be able to have my grandmother living with us over those many years, despite the difficulties and frustrations. I know not everyone is in a position to do that.

Anne's Story

The force that held my mum stable and calm was the undying love Dad had for her. He was amazing, though sorely tested, and, in the end, he needed full-time help. We found a care home for Mum, and then Dad followed shortly after so that they could be together but be cared for individually. The staff were so lovely, and the cultural backgrounds they came from created a warm, respectful environment where nothing was too difficult to manage and where faith in God was not a foreign concept. We were so grateful. By now Mum was so advanced in her dementia that I needed to focus my attention on Dad, who felt the loneliness of being a widower-in-waiting keenly. He had spent so much time on the sidelines, supporting Mum; he seemed depleted. I wanted, more than anything, to remind him of how wonderful he was and to show how much he was loved by Mum, by each of his children and grandchildren and especially by me. He had shown all of us the love that Jesus had inspired in him. We wanted to reflect that love back to him.

Day 30

The Last Word

After you have suffered a little while, the God of all grace, who has called you to his eternal glory in Christ, will himself restore, confirm, strengthen and establish you.

1 Peter 5:10

Suffering is part of our life in a fallen world. God doesn't promise to take us out of it, but as we have seen, he promises to be with us in it. His presence gives us hope now, as well as for the future.

Peter's readers were facing suffering and pressure. He refers to this throughout his letter, and here, at the end, he gives an astonishing promise: God will "*himself* restore, confirm, strengthen and establish you". "Himself" is as emphatic in the original language as it is in translation. It's worth unpacking this promise.

First, *suffering is assumed*. We don't come out of it; we come through it. Emily realised this as she read from Isaiah after her husband, David, was diagnosed: "Fear not, for I have redeemed you; I have called you by name, you are mine. When you pass through the waters, I will be with you" (Isaiah 43:1-2). The word to note here is "when". These trials will come, but he promises to be with us.

The God who brings us through always shows us an *attitude of grace,* accepting us despite our faltering efforts to serve and to love. We are conscious of the things we could and should have done better. We wish we could have done more. But he doesn't deal with us as we deserve. Instead, he *promises us a great future*, secure in his eternal purpose—and full of glory.

And our God will *personally make sure* that we are cared for: that we know we are loved and that he is working for us. In the end, we will find that the days and years which we thought we had lost have not been wasted. He will give us back more, though our experience of suffering will have left its mark. We will be scarred, but our character will have been tested and shaped to be more like Jesus, and our faith will be strengthened. He promises to "restore, confirm, strengthen and establish" us. It is a comprehensive restoration.

As we care for somebody, along with all the challenges, we can experience an intense relationship, with its own joy. In the same way, we can find an intense awareness of God's presence with us through all that we are experiencing: times of testing as well as finding him faithful. These are significant and precious experiences of his love and care—sometimes when we are alone, sometimes with others or perhaps in church. This is our God *himself,* who is with us.

This is the heart of all these reflections. You can look back over these devotions and pick out the aspects of God's character and promises that stood out for you. For me, I love the picture of the strong tower into which I can run (Proverbs 18:10, Day 2), or the reassurance that I have been engraved on his palms (Isaiah 49:16, Day 9), or the promise of going home to be with him for ever (John 14:3, Day 19).

Our God has promised to be with us himself, all the way through. Sometimes we may feel—like Betty Davis, who cared for her husband, Robert—that he is holding us "in that special place of all who are called to share 'the fellowship of his suffering'".[59]

Even then, as we call out, "How long, O Lord?" we still say:

But I trust in your unfailing love. (Psalm 13:1, 5)

Reflect

Look again at the reflections and stories that have meant the most to you. What truths about God have you learned or remembered afresh? Make a note of some of the things that have challenged you most and encouraged you most.

Appendix

Responding to Dementia: Helpful Books and Resources

Here are some of the books that I found most helpful at our most challenging time and since then.

You can also find many resources at AlzAuthors (alzauthors.com), who have a growing collection of books, articles, podcasts and resources, from the USA and other countries, including many personal stories.

Simple introductions

John Zeisel, *I'm Still Here,* (Piatkus, 2011)
The person with Alzheimer's is still the same person with whom we can relate, but it is a different relationship. That is the main point of this warm and beautifully written book. It also gives a basic understanding of Alzheimer's and its main symptoms and their effects, together with detailed practical guidelines for communicating and building the new relationship.

This was the first book I read at a time when I was struggling to understand what was happening. It was a revelation, giving a clear and sympathetic understanding of the person living with Alzheimer's.

John Dunlop, *Finding Grace in the Face of Dementia*, (Crossway, 2017)

I read this book later than Zeisel's, but I would put it in equal place at the head of the list. It gives a clear and warm introduction to the medical facts, along with practical advice on how to relate and care. Dunlop's position as a geriatric physician gives authority to the medical part, while his experience of caring for his own parents makes his practical advice compassionate and authentic.

William Cutting, *Dementia: A Positive Response*, (Onwards and Upwards, 2018)

Good medical material with a lot of practical advice. It covers similar ground to the other introductions. Dr Cutting especially advocates a very positive and active response to the early stages, in the conviction that this will help people to lead a full and even comfortable life.

Simon Atkins, *First Steps to Living with Dementia*, (Lion Hudson, 2013)

Written by a doctor; another clear and sympathetic overview, from medical facts to practical responses. Quite brief, so easy to digest!

Tina English: *A Great Place to Grow Old*, (Darton, Longman & Todd, 2021)
A simple and accessible introduction to working with older people in general. The chapter on dementia gives a clear and comprehensive overview in just 20 pages, while the next chapter on carers is helpful in examining the challenges that carers face and gives some resources for supporting them.

Lee-Fay Low, *Live and Laugh with Dementia*, (Exisle Publishing, 2014)
This has a simple focus: how to maintain active relationships with the person living with dementia. It is extremely practical and full of optimism, with fascinating case studies of people at different stages of dementia, enabling you to assess what stage your situation has reached. I wish I had read this sooner.

Stephen Miller, *Communicating Across Dementia*, (Robinson, 2015)
Clear guidance on how to talk, listen, provide stimulation and give comfort to people living with dementia. The author covers almost all the relevant areas in a sensitive way, turning some of the key principles that other books advocate into simple and practical guidelines, with many examples.

Personal stories

Sally Magnusson, *Where Memories Go*, (Two Roads, 2014)
The story of her mother, Mamie: her gradual descent into Alzheimer's and the struggles of her children as they cared

for her. The detailed accounts of their actual situation and the gaps in the system rang true to our experience. I kept nodding, "Yes, just like us," and was eager to learn what happened next.

Oliver James, *Contented Dementia*, (Vermilion, 2009)

This is based on the story of Penny Garton caring for her mother, which is the starting point for a much wider exploration and definite guidelines for supporting people with dementia. It is a very particular approach. Some of it was less applicable to me, but the main thesis was really helpful: the person with dementia needs to be respected within their present world and frame of reference. So don't keep asking questions; learn from them—enter into their world.

Robertson McQuilkin, *A Promise Kept*, (Tyndale House Publishers, 1999)

A remarkable short story of faithfulness and love, caring for his wife for 25 years. Very inspiring.

Christine Bryden, *Who will I be when I die?* (Jessica Kingsley Publishers, 1998, 2012)

Christine Bryden was a high-flying government official in her 50s when she was diagnosed with young-onset dementia in 1995. She describes vividly the shock of her early experiences of dementia, her work for advocacy and the measure of healing she has also experienced, through the prayer of many friends. A second edition, sixteen years after her diagnosis, marks her continuing life with dementia.

Christine Bryden, *Dancing with Dementia*, (Jessica Kingsley Publishers, 2005)
This continues Christine's story of living positively with dementia, helping to bring radical change in understanding and attitudes to people living with dementia. It contains more detail of what it is like to live with dementia, her fears of losing her identity and her trust in God for the present and future. Both books are remarkable accounts of faith and hope.

Jennifer Bute with Louise Morse, *Dementia From the Inside: A Doctor's Personal Journey of Hope*, (SPCK, 2018)
Jennifer Bute's experience of early-onset dementia enables her to speak "from the inside"—to show the many positive aspects, in contrast to common fears and stereotypes. As with Christine Bryden and Wendy Mitchell's books, her insights are valuable for caregivers and families too.

Robin Thomson, *Living with Alzheimer's—A Love Story*, (Instant Apostle, 2020)
My personal story of receiving Shoko's diagnosis of Alzheimer's disease. We learned the hard way, going through relentless pressure as Shoko's personality gradually changed and she lost her capacity in many areas—but not her constant affection and love. We also experienced love and practical help from family and friends, backed up by health and social care professionals.

Wendy Mitchell, *Somebody I Used to Know*, (Bloomsbury, 2019)
The writer was diagnosed in 2014 as having young-onset Alzheimer's, at the age of 58. She wrote and spoke all over

the country about her condition, giving a remarkable picture from the inside. Although she and others like her are a minority, their insights are really valuable for families and caregivers.

Wendy Mitchell, *What I Wish People Knew About Dementia, From Someone Who Knows,* **(Bloomsbury, 2022)**
Described as a "practical guide to living with dementia". It took Wendy "many years to work out strategies that enabled her to 'live well with dementia' … Her book is a compilation of these strategies: a kind of how-to manual for people with the condition and those who support them." (Review by author Nicci Gerrard in the *Guardian*, Tuesday 1 February, 2022)

Jude Wilton, *Can I Tell You About Dementia? A Guide for Family, Friends and Carers,* **(Jessica Kingsley Publishers, 2013)**
This isn't really a story, but it comes through the words of "Jack", a person living with dementia, describing his experience, which gives the basis for simple, practical and encouraging advice.

Lucy Whitman (editor), *Telling Tales About Dementia,* **(Jessica Kingsley Publishers, 2010)**
A collection of 30 stories by those caring for a parent, partner or friend with dementia. They reflect on their experiences of pain and loss, the struggles with finding support, and the hope and love that they also discovered. The whole book is moving and informative.

Adam Sibley, *Unbreakable Bond*, (TeamSibley Publishing, 2015)
Adam Sibley was 25 when he began caring for his mother, who was diagnosed with young-onset dementia when she was 51. He tells very simply what it was like, giving practical advice and insight for anybody called to the same experience.

Some comprehensive perspectives

Julian Hughes, *Alzheimer's and Other Dementias (The Facts)*, (Oxford University Press, 2011)
Fairly short but remarkably detailed and authoritative, with good material on the personal and spiritual care of people with dementia.

June Andrews, *Dementia: The One-Stop Guide*, (Profile Books, 2015)
This is comprehensive, as its title suggests, covering the medical, social, practical, financial and legal aspects. That means that some parts are brief, but it's a reliable overall guide.

Bernard Coope and Felicity Richards (editors), *ABC of Dementia*, (Wiley-Blackwell, 2007)
This is written for doctors and other medical personnel, so it is quite technical in parts. It covers all areas, with strong sections on person-centred care and the use and limitations of medication.

Reflections and further resources

John Killick, *Dementia Positive*, (Luath Press Limited, 2014)
The subtitle is *A Handbook Based on Lived Experiences*. John Killick has worked with people with dementia and their carers for many years. He shares their experiences, often in their own words, to show creative ways in which we can relate to people with dementia. Accessible, practical and positive.

John Swinton, *Dementia: Living in the Memories of God*, (SCM Press, 2012)
A reflection on what it means to be a person in the context of a disease which takes away memory and threatens self-consciousness. Definitely not an introductory book but deep and ultimately very encouraging. It particularly brings out the importance of community and friendship to sustain relationships with those living with dementia.

Joanna Collicutt, *Thinking of You: A Resource for the Spiritual Care of People with Dementia*, (Bible Reading Fellowship, 2017)
A comprehensive introduction: dementia itself and its medical and social effects; what happens to the person living with dementia, in relation to themselves, to others and to God; and spiritual care. The final section has guidelines for dementia-friendly churches.

Nicci Gerrard, *What Dementia Teaches us about Love*, (Allen Lane, 2019)
The author reflects on her relationship with her father, who died from dementia. This led her to interview people of

all backgrounds—those living with dementia, caregivers, health and social care professionals, researchers—searching for answers to the deep questions and truths that dementia raises for us as individuals and as a society.

Louise Morse, *Worshipping with Dementia*, (Monarch Books, 2010)

People living with dementia are still people who can connect spiritually at deep levels. A collection of meditations, Bible passages, prayers and hymns for caregivers, people living with dementia, families, church groups and medical or social care professionals. Its simplicity is its great strength.

Tricia Williams, *What Happens to Faith when Christians Get Dementia?* (Pickwick Publications, 2021)

An in-depth qualitative study of four men and four women living with mild to moderate dementia. "The main thrust of the book is that the engrained faith experience gained in earlier years and from belonging to a faith community can continue into the later stages of dementia and even go on growing. The writer makes pertinent recommendations for the local church, the wider community of faith and the development of new theological perspectives." (From a review in the Dementia Newsletter No. 57, May 2021.)

Wendy Gleadle and Frances Attwood, *Dementia, God and the Church: Journeying with Hope*, (Bible Reading Fellowship, 2026—forthcoming)

A positive response: faith is not simply cognitive but an expression of the whole person, so those living with dementia can still communicate with God even when their cognition declines. God continues to communicate with them. The church has a vital role to support families affected by dementia.

There are many more books, articles and other resources on every aspect of dementia. You will find references in the books listed above. I have not included any of those that give advice on diet, exercise and lifestyle, nor those explaining research into the causes and possible cures, except this:

Joseph Jebelli, *In Pursuit of Memory*, (John Murray, 2017)
A brilliant survey exploring the many different avenues in the search for causes and cures for Alzheimer's, from Alois Alzheimer in 1906 up to the time of publication. Since then there have been a number of significant advances in medication. The research continues.

Some helpful websites and organisations

AlzAuthors | alzauthors.com
A network of publications and resources from the USA.

Alzheimer's Disease International | www.alzint.org
"The Global Voice on Dementia" supports and works with Alzheimer's and dementia associations in 120 countries, as well as people living with dementia, carers, and all relevant organisations. Its aim is to help raise awareness, challenge stigma and to call for dementia to be the global health priority it needs to be.

Alzheimer's Society or Association | www.alz.org (USA) | www.alzheimers.org.uk (UK)
Gives comprehensive information and links for many different countries.

Being Patient | beingpatient.com
Covering the latest Alzheimer's and dementia news through journalism, patient perspectives and exclusive interviews with leading experts. News, advice, stories and support.

Dementia Network Newsletter
Twice-yearly newsletter with helpful information, book reviews and comments, produced by Christians on Ageing. Email info@ccoa.org.uk or visit christiansonageing.org.uk.

Embracing Age | www.embracingage.org.uk
Christian charity working towards a world where older people are valued, connected and full of hope, by combatting loneliness, mobilising volunteers and equipping churches.

Faith in Later Life | faithinlaterlife.org
Faith in Later Life inspires and equips Christians to reach, serve and empower older people through the local church.

Legal and financial questions

Pathways Through Dementia
pathwaysthroughdementia.org
Provides free, accurate legal and financial information to support people living with dementia.

Livability | www.livability.org.uk
Christian charity that's committed to enabling people with disabilities to live the life they want to lead. Excellent material on how churches can welcome and be inclusive.

WHO iSupport manual
www.who.int/publications/i/item/9789241515863
An online knowledge and skills training programme—a self-help tool for carers of people with dementia, including family members, relatives and friends. Available online or as printed pdf. Five modules with accompanying exercises.

Examples of church initiatives

Anna Chaplains | www.annachaplaincy.org.uk
Offering spiritual care in later life:
www.annachaplaincy.org.uk/dementia-resources

Caraway | www.caraway.uk.com
"Spiritually resourcing the older person." Working together with the local church and the health and social sectors in Southampton.

Caring for Caregivers and Building Support Teams
www.embracingage.org.uk/supporting-carers-course.html
Free training material for churches to support those living with dementia.

The Crowborough Barnabas Support Group
www.allsaintscrowborough.org

Endnotes

1. Robin Thomson, *Living with Alzheimer's—A Love Story* (Instant Apostle, 2020) https://instantapostle.com/books/living-with-alzheimers/

2. There are many summaries of what dementia is. This comes from Alzheimer's Disease International (https://www.alzint.org/about/): "Dementia is an umbrella term for a collection of symptoms that are caused by disorders affecting the brain and impact on memory, thinking, behaviour and emotion. The most common is Alzheimer's disease, which affects 50-60% of people with dementia. Other types of dementia include vascular dementia, Lewy body dementia and fronto-temporal dementia." There are up to 100 different types.

3. Claire Webster, Serge Gauthier, "Impact of the Diagnosis on Carers", World Alzheimer Report 2022, Alzheimer's Disease International, p. 72 https://www.alzint.org/resource/world-alzheimer-report-2022/ (accessed 10 October 2024).

4. Wendy Mitchell, *Somebody I Used to Know* (Bloomsbury Publishing, 2018).

5. John McArthur, *Philippians: The MacArthur New Testament Commentary* (Moody Publishers, 1995) p. 296.

6. Lewis de Marolles, "An Essay on Providence", translated from the French by John Martin, 1790, p. 42.

7   From a poem by Betty Scott Stam, missionary in China, martyred there with her husband, John, in 1937. https://library.timelesstruths.org/texts/Foundation_Truth_7/In_the_Center_of_the_Circle/ https://www.reviveourhearts.com/blog/betty-scott-stam-life-surrender/ (accessed 7 August 2024).

8   John Dunlop, *Finding Grace in the Face of Dementia* (Crossway, 2017).

9   "Glorious Things of Thee Are Spoken", John Newton, 1779.

10 Federico Villanueva, *It's OK to Be Not OK: Preaching the Lament Psalms* (Langham Preaching Resources, 2017).

11 John Zeisel, *I'm Still Here* (Piatkus, 2011).

12 Jackie Macadam, "Interview with Mary Warnock: 'A Duty to Die?'", *Life and Work*, October 2008, p. 25. Quoted in John Swinton, *Dementia: Living in the Memories of God* (SCM Press, 2nd edition, 2017) p. 121.

13 John Swinton, *Dementia: Living in the Memories of God* (SCM Press, 2nd edition, 2017) p. 283-284.

14 John Killick, *Dementia Positive* (Luath Press Limited, 2014), p. 95-101.

15 Tom Kitwood, *Dementia Reconsidered: The Person Comes First* (Open University Press, 1997, p. 58-64.

16 Kitwood, p. 80-84.

17   Zelda Freitas, "Navigating the Carer Journey as a Daughter and Social Worker", World Alzheimer Report 2022, Alzheimer's Disease International, p. 266 https://www.alzint.org/resource/world-alzheimer-report-2022/ (accessed 7 August, 2024).

18   "Anna Chaplains" provide spiritual care and emotional and spiritual support for older people www.annachaplaincy.org.uk.

19   Robert Davis, *My Journey into Alzheimer's Disease* (Tyndale House, 1989), p. 53.

20   Swinton, p. 284.

21   Swinton, p. 193-198, 222-223.

22   Christine Bryden, Elizabeth McKinlay, *Dementia: A Spiritual Journey Towards the Divine*, quoted in Swinton, p. 193.

23   Teepa Snow, at a conference in June 2019. See also teepasnow.com.

24   Robertson McQuilkin, *A Promise Kept* (Tyndale House Publishers, 1999).

25   Psalms 3, 7, 18, 34, 51, 52, 54, 56, 57, 59, 60, 63, 142.

26   Gordon Wenham, *The Psalter Reclaimed* (Crossway, 2013), p. 69.

27   Christopher Wright, quoted in Federico Villanueva, *It's OK to Be Not OK: Preaching the Lament Psalms*, p. xiv.

28   Wenham, p. 44.

29 Villanueva, p. 123.

30 Villanueva, p. 124.

31 Christopher Wright, Villanueva, p. xiv.

32 www.sportskeeda.com/tennis/when-i-holding-cup-i-never-asked-god-why-me-arthur-ashe-s-emotional-letter-fan-last-days (accessed 7 August 2024).

33 Arthur Ashe, Arnold Rampesaud, *Days of Grace* (Ballantine Books, 1993), p. 326.

34 Dunlop, p. 157.

35 Christine Bryant, "Let's talk about having dementia", *Dancing with Dementia* (Jessica Kingsley Publishers, 2005), p. 102-114.

36 Michael Horton, in Nancy Guthrie, *O Love That Will Not Let Me Go* (Crossway, 2011), p. 19-26.

37 Nicci Gerrard, *What Dementia Teaches Us About Love* (Allen Lane, 2017), p. 220, 221.

38 Edward Shillito, *Jesus of the Scars: And Other Poems* (Hodder and Stoughton, 1919).

39 www.alzheimers.org.uk/about-dementia/symptoms-and-diagnosis/symptoms/sundowning (accessed 7 August 2024).

40 See especially Tom Kitwood, *Rethinking Dementia* and John Zeisel, *I'm Still Here.*

41 Christine Bryden, "Who will I be when I die?", p. 120-126; *Dancing with Dementia,* p. 175-181

42   Christine Bryden, Elizabeth MacKinlay, "Dementia: a Spiritual Journey Towards the Divine: A Personal View of Dementia", *Journal of Religious Gerontology 13,* Issues 3 & 4, 2003, p. 72, 73. Quoted in Swinton, p. 193-94 (including quotation from Christine Bryden, *Dancing with Dementia* (Jessica Kingsley Publishers, 2005).

43   Facebook post, September 2023, used by permission.

44   Facebook post, January 2022, used by permission.

45   "My Friend Suri Williams, A Tribute by Ajith Fernando, 15th January 2018", email 15 January 2018.

46   Mitchell, *Somebody I Used to Know*, p. 138.

47   Quoted in Swinton, p. 193-94.

48   Gerrard, p. 232-233.

49   Frank Houghton, *Amy Carmichael of Dohnavur* (SPCK, 1956) p. 358.

50   Adam Sibley, *Unbreakable Bond* (TeamSibley Publishing, 2015), p. 19.

51   Ajith Fernando, email 24 January 2017.

52   Kitwood, p. 43.

53   Christine Bryden's "Letter to the Church", *Journal of Disability and Religion, Vol. 22,* p. 96-106.

54   Christine Bryden, *Dancing with Dementia,* p. 150.

55   Sally Magnusson, *Where Memories Go* (Two Roads, 2014), p. 298.

56   Swinton, p. 180.

57   Swinton, p. 181.

58   Christine Bryden, *Dancing with Dementia*, p. 110.

59   Robert Davis, p.139.

thegoodbook
COMPANY

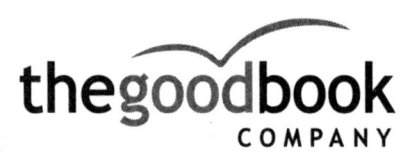

BIBLICAL | RELEVANT | ACCESSIBLE

At The Good Book Company we are dedicated to helping Christians and local churches grow. We believe that God's growth process always starts with hearing clearly what he has said to us through his timeless and flawless word—the Bible.

Ever since we opened our doors in 1991, we have been striving to produce resources that are biblical, relevant, and accessible. By God's grace, we have grown to become an international publisher, encouraging ordinary Christians of every age and stage and every background and denomination to live for Christ day by day and equipping churches to grow in their knowledge of God, their love for one another, and the effectiveness of their outreach.

Call one of our friendly team for a discussion of your needs or visit one of our local websites for more information on the resources and services we provide.

Your friends at The Good Book Company

thegoodbook.com | thegoodbook.co.uk
thegoodbook.com.au | thegoodbook.co.nz